From FAT to SLIM in 3 Steps!

Providing Help For Your Journey From Fat Land to Slim Land

The Strategic Way to achieve Long Term Successful Weight Control and develop the Positive Lifestyle Management skills required to reach and then to stay in Slim Land and live a happy life.

An original work by

Guru David

aka David John Sheridan

A weight problem is a set of conditions and circumstances looking for a better way of being understood and managed. We use work from The Human Algorithm® Project to do this.

For the 84% or more of dieters who normally fail on diets.

Published by Sheridan Publishing in July 2015

Previously published by Amazon in 2014

Updated in May 2021

ISBN 978-0-9932355-2-8

DEDICATION

I dedicate this book to my cousin and childhood friend who recently died: Mr Bernard Balzanelli.

A part of a family, the Balzanelli's, which it has been my pleasure to know for all of my life.

Go Bernard!

From Fat to Slim in 3 Steps

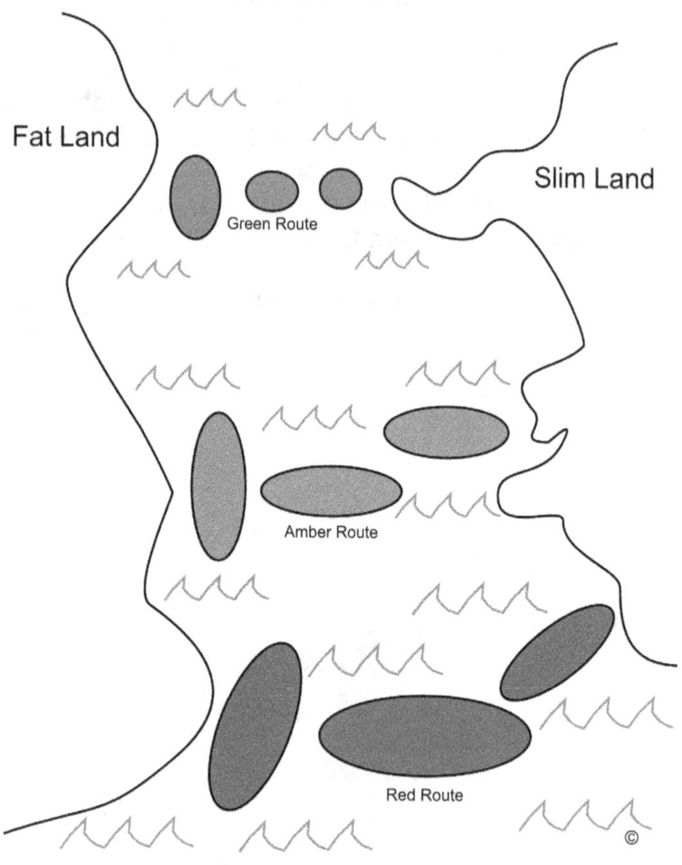

The Journey from Fat Land to Slim Land

Make your way across the Stepping Stones with different challenges and obstacles to overcome along the way.

Then you need to learn how to stay in Slim Land with the help of The Human Algorithm® Project.

Books by this Author include:

For Adults

Weight Control The Hi-Way

From FAT To SLIM In 3 Steps

The Perfect Life Diet For Imperfect People With Weight Problems

Motivate & Inspire Yourself; To Do Something Positive

Self-Esteem For Imperfect People

An Introduction To The Human Dynamics Matrix

For Children

The Magic Mustachio and the tale of The Bear That Loved Pies

CONTENTS

ACKNOWLEDGMENTS

Tempus Fugit

Time Flies

Intellectual Property Rights

This work is an Application of The Human Algorithm® project which was invented and developed by David John Sheridan aka Guru David.

The Human Algorithm® is a Platform for understanding and working with any type of problem which involves Human Behaviour; in personal, professional and business situations.

This book and its contents are an Application of this Platform for people with persistent weight problems and weight management problems. It has been designed to help them improve, resolve and better manage their persistent weight problem and to improve their overall quality of life.

INTRODUCTION

In this book I will introduce you to a new and effective approach to losing weight and successfully managing your weight over the long term.

I will show you how to become successful at managing your weight long term and how to improve your life along the way.

There is no calorie counting, there are no foods that you can't eat, there is no potion control, there are no diet products that you need to purchase or use and there are no fad diets.

What we have here is a process that really works and which changes and improves people's lives.

We are going to be working with the actual structure (the architecture) of weight problems and changing that structure so that you no longer have the problem.

This can give you Mastery over your weight problem and help you to achieve the lifestyle that you really want to have.

I have written this book so that it is accessible to everyone with a persistent weight problem. You don't need any special skills or abilities. All you need to be able to do is to understand the difference between Red, Amber and Green.

I will help you to understand what type of weight problem you actually have and we will use The Dieters Scale© to do this.

Unusually for a diet book; this book can be used by people who are underweight as well as those who are overweight.

All the principles apply to both groups and they both have the same question: how does someone get to a target weight and maintain that weight over the long term?

I am going to introduce you to The Stepping Stones Approach. And in the Stepping Stones Approach it doesn't matter what your previous dieting history is like.

It doesn't matter whether you are a seasoned dieter or someone who is about to undertake your first diet; this approach can help you.

It also doesn't matter whether you are a little overweight or a lot overweight; The Human Algorithm® Stepping Stones Approach will apply to you and you can use it to achieve positive results that can be sustained.

With this approach it also doesn't matter what diet you want to use; or, whether you are going to an organised slimming club or doing it on your own. The principles of The Human Algorithm® Stepping Stones Approach apply in all cases.

This means that you can go to a slimming club and use The Stepping Stones approach; but you need to separate out what I am saying from what they are saying; and don't let yourself get confused or let yourself be taken in the wrong direction.

What you need to remember about slimming clubs and dieting organisations is that they have a very high long term failure rates. As much as 84% of their members fail each year.

With The Stepping Stones Approach I want to speak to that 84% who normally fail. I want to help them to do a better job and achieve better results that can last longer; hopefully for a lifetime.

So if you use a slimming club or weight watching club, you need to understand their limitations and their business focus.

Try to look at the results that they really do actually achieve over the long term for most of their members; and don't let yourself get distracted by the marketing hype that focuses on what only a few people achieve.

In The Stepping Stones Approach it doesn't matter whether you can exercise or not. Exercise is not required as part of losing weight and keeping weight off.

You can think of The Stepping Stones Approach as being a Strategic Journey that you will undertake to improve your life and achieve a lifestyle that you are happy with.

We don't want you to be a super model, we want you to reach your "happy point" and to be happy with whom and how you are.

On this journey you may encounter wrong turns; and you may become stuck on a particular Stepping Stone or fall off the Stepping Stones altogether. If this happens it doesn't matter because this is life and this is what happens in life. You learn from mistakes and poor choices and you correct them.

To overcome these problem you simply start the Stepping Stones Approach from the beginning once more and learn from what you have already done.

In the Stepping Stones Approach we believe that practice makes perfect and that it's OK to make mistakes when you practice. It's what practice is for!

Using this simple approach, you will know which Stepping Stone you are on at any time; and you will know what you need to do to stay on it and progress forwards towards Slim Land.

If you do have a problem, you will also know which Stepping Stone you have fallen off or tried to skip over, to try and get into Slim Land faster.

Falling off a Stepping Stone is not a problem. Failure doesn't matter in this process, because failure is simply part of the journey to success that you need to undertake to get to where you want to be: Slim Land.

When you have had enough of failure, you will then take the time and put in the appropriate effort to complete the Stepping Stones journey in the right way.

If you try to rush through the 3 steps and get to the end result; then you are likely to fail and have to begin again.

> You won't be able to stay in Slim Land if you cheat, because all you are doing in cheating yourself. So if you win by cheating you actually lose!

If you fall off the 1st, 2nd or 3rd Stepping Stones, all you need to do is go back to the start and begin the process once more. Don't try and start from anywhere other than the beginning because it won't work well.

If you try to jump from one Stepping Stone to another too quickly; then you are likely to fall off. This is because you are not doing what needs to be done to achieve and maintain what you are after; living in Slim Land.

It really doesn't matter whether you need to go through The Stepping Stones Approach once or a number of times before you get it right; whatever it takes for you is what is acceptable and OK.

This is a personal challenge that you will undertake!

Some people may use The Stepping Stones Approach a number of times. Each time they will move closer and closer to being able to live in Slim Land.

It is perfectly acceptable to use this baby steps approach when you are learning from each attempt and you progress slowly forwards.

It is also in the nature of journeys that sometimes we need to go backwards to enable us to progress further forwards.

Your journey from Fat Land to Slim Land can also follow this same path. And if it does; do not worry because this approach has been designed to deal with that.

Taking a bit longer to get to Slim Land usually produces better and more sustainable results than going at it too fast.

There is no point trying to be competitive with The Stepping Stones Approach. You can do so but then you may not do things in the way that you personally need to do them in order to get to Slim Land. As a result you may fall off a Stepping Stone and find yourself back in Fat Land.

You may come across someone who claims that they have short cuts and they know simple ways to cross the Stepping Stones.

In reality the people who keep looking for quick fixes and easy ways; often end up doing things the hard way and not achieving what they really want. Why waste time and effort when you can use them in a positive way?

Your destiny is in the Stepping Stones and you need to fulfil your destiny. To do this you need to undertake the journey.

The Stepping Stones Approach is really about you. Not anyone else; just you!

You see I could work with 100 people and each one will need to do things at the pace that is right for them and in the way that is right for them.

It doesn't matter that I could push them to do things faster and to lose weight quicker. You see what I am after is successful long term results that you can build on and develop further.

I am not interested in the short term results that cannot be sustained and which fall away quickly; leaving you disappointed and worse off than before.

What you need to understand is that most dieters who use normal diets and diet products fall off and fail on the 1st and 2nd Stepping Stones.

This is because they try to jump straight on to the 2nd Stepping Stone (Dieting) and from there they try to jump into Slim Land.

It becomes like one of those obstacle courses you see on television where people keep getting knocked into the water despite their efforts. Splash! Back to Fat Land.

Most dieters are never told about the 1st and the 3rd Stepping Stones.

As a result most dieters try to jump from Fat Land on to the 2nd Stepping Stone (Dieting), and from there they try to jump over the 3rd Stepping Stone and into Slim Land.

No wonder so many of them fail because the distances are too great to do this. It just can't be done by most people.

In reality conventional dieting and the different diet plans and dieting organisations have a real big problem: The solutions that they sell have so much failure attached to them.

84% of the people who diet fail.

If you want to be successful then you need to do something different from what you have done in the past.

With The Stepping Stones Approach we can make good use of any failure that you experience and turn it into something useful; rather than something which makes us feel bad.

We can turn the negative into something positive:

Knowledge!

We can turn your failure into Knowledge because we can use your "failure experiences" as an opportunity to learn and do something different in the future.

Rather than throw our toys out of the pram, let's be adults and accept that this is a tough thing to do and that problems do occur when you do tough things.

The Stepping Stones Approach really isn't afraid of failure; because for 84% of dieters failure is a reality of their normal dieting experiences and their lives.

We need to embrace failure and use it as a guide to achieving success.

Failure is showing us that we are not doing the right

things, in the right way, for the right reason; at the right time!

The Stepping Stones Approach to dieting, slimming and long term weight control has been developed by me; David John Sheridan, using work from The Human Algorithm® Project.

We have now combined this work into The Human Algorithm® Project and this has been developed further into Weight Control The Hi-Waynny approach to persistent weight problems.

So without further ado: Let's begin your journey from Fat Land to Slim Land in 3 Steps!

Read through the whole book first and then begin working through it.

If you jump sections and ignore sections then you will probably fail.

Keep the book available so that you can make sure that you are doing the right things and to avoid getting seduced by the marketing promises of the Dieting, Beauty and Health industries.

Many people may try to take you off the path and try to keep you in Fat Land; don't let them do it.

The only person that you really need to be on your side so that you will succeed; is you!

Reaching The 1st Stepping Stone!

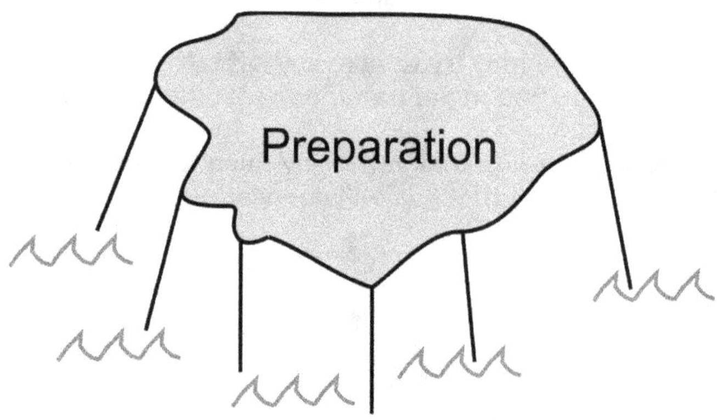

CHAPTER 1

The 1st Stepping Stone

The 1st Stepping Stone that you need to reach is called Preparation.

At the moment you are stuck in a place which we will call "Fat Land".

To get out of Fat Land and into Slim Land you need to cross The 3 Stepping Stones.

Along the way there are going to be challenges and victories. Some things you will find easy and some things will be harder; but if you keep going you will get to Slim Land.

If you fall off The Stepping Stones then you go back to Fat Land. If you rush across The Stepping Stones to get into Slim Land; then you will wake up one day and find yourself back in Fat Land.

If you try and cheat to get to Slim Land then the same thing will happen; you just simply won't be able to stay there and you will find yourself back in Fat Land.

So are you ready to begin your quest?

You are going to undertake a journey from Fat Land to Slim Land. And like all journeys; it's the experiences that you have along the way that really count.

So what do you need to do before you can reach that 1st Stepping Stone?

First you need to understand what part of Fat Land you are actually living in; and what type of journey you actually need to undertake to get out of there.

You see Fat Land has a landscape which contains different Zones. The terrain in those different zones varies and travelling to Slim Land from those different Zones becomes increasingly difficult.

The different Zones are Green, Amber and Red.

> A Green Zone is easier to navigate than the Amber Zone.
>
> An Amber Zone is easier to navigate than the Red Zone.
>
> A Red Zone is the most difficult to navigate.

As a result of these different Zones (and the various obstacles in them) people need to go by different routes to get out of Fat Land and into Slim Land.

They can't all go by the same route!

To help us understand where you are living in Fat Land and to help us work out what route you need to take to get to Slim Land, we will use and apply The Dieters Scale©™.

The Dieters Scale is a simple process that I created and it helps us to see how difficult your problem really is and whereabouts in Fat Land you are actually living.

You might be living in an easy Zone or a more difficult Zone. We need to find that out first as it affects the route you will need to take.

What we need to know is: Do you need to use the Green route, the Amber route or the Red route?

From Fat to Slim in 3 Steps

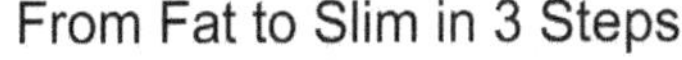

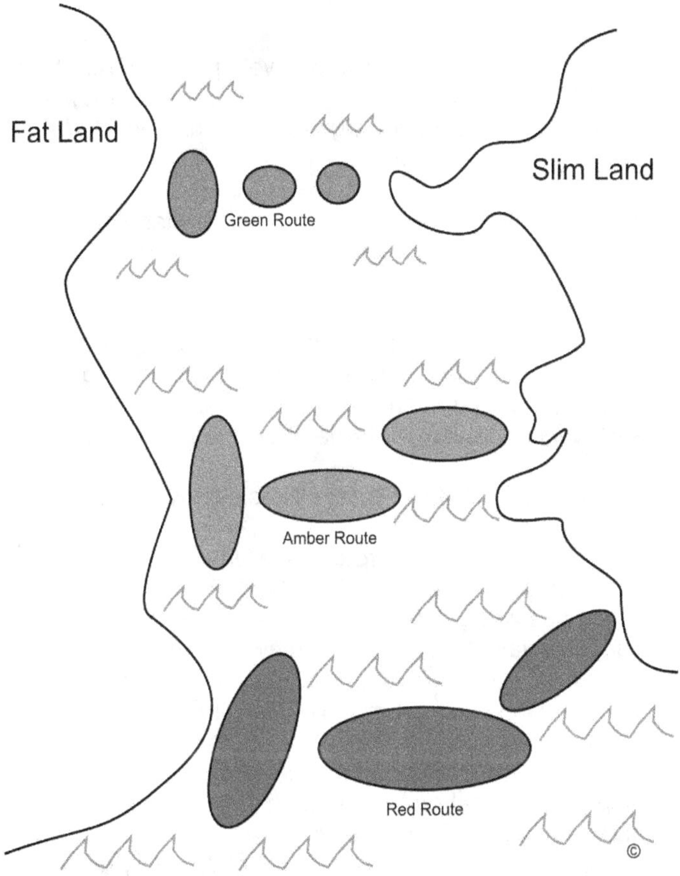
Fat Land
Slim Land
Green Route
Amber Route
Red Route
©

CHAPTER 2

Where Are You On The Dieters Scale?

When I work with people who have a problem with their weight; I find that they can have a lot of confusion and uncertainty about their weight problem and how to deal with it.

This is usually caused by a lack of understanding, inappropriate information and having the wrong expectations.

What also causes a great deal of confusion and uncertainty, is the media and the constant focus of certain publications and programmes about what someone looks like; and what they should look like.

On top of this we have things like celebrity diets.

In another book that I wrote (The Perfect Life Diet For Imperfect People With Weight Problems) I look at celebrities who put on weight, lose weight, put on weight and lose weight. They make an awful lot of money from selling one diet plan after another; and many of them make a career out of being Yo-Yo dieters.

I have to say that none of these celebrities seems to help with the real problem of long term weight control and helping people with moving away from dieting; and becoming someone who used to diet. But they do drag a lot of good people into bad dieting habits and into having the wrong expectations of what a diet can deliver and how easy and simple it all is.

In all things there is a right way to do something and a wrong way. Following these fad diet processes and hoping that they can take you to the promised land, keep you slim and help you to stay slim; is usually a folly. These are false gods that make you worship at the altar of false promises and unattainable results.

Let's accept that you are probably one of the 84% of normal dieters who fail with diets and managing your weight. And so let's work from that position without any false promises or claims.

You are living in Fat Land and you would prefer to live in Slim Land but you can't get there; so let me help you with that.

Let's just deal with the real problems and move it along without getting distracted.

As part of my work of developing solutions to problems that involve people; I look at the structure and nature of problems. This helps me to see and understand what I am really working with.

It is not unusual for me to find that the real problem, the thing that is actually causing the problem, is actually different from the problem someone thought that they had.

With dieting, slimming and long term weight control I have found the same thing. People are often trying to fix the wrong things in the wrong ways.

What I see is that most dieters are applying a solution to their weight problem that isn't capable of really fixing it.

With so many people who diet there is a mismatch between their weight problem and the dieting solution that they are trying to use to fix it.

> Do you think that this mismatching contributes to the 84% failure rate that dieters have?

To help me understand the problems that people have with their weight in a better way; and to help me sort things out so that I could work with them better; I began actually looking at weight problems in different ways.

In reality; different people have different types of weight problems.

So how do you know what type of weight problem you have?

People use things like the Body Mass Index (BMI) and percentage of body fat, etc. But in my experience none of these are really impacting weight problems in the right way.

The truth is that more people are developing persistent weight problems and it is a growing trend for us to have more obese people and more morbidly obese people.

To help to change this trend I needed to do something different to what other people were doing!

To help me sort out the different types of weight problems, so that they could be worked with more effectively; I created and developed a number of different tools. One of those tools is The Dieters Scale©.

The purpose behind The Dieters Scale© is that it allows us, you and me, to begin to see and understand the structure and nature of any weight problem.

Once we know what this structure is, we can then design and develop the proper type of solution to improve, resolve or better manage it.

It's simple really: Square pegs go into square hole and not into round holes. Dieters are putting the wrong pegs into the wrong holes and they have been doing so for many years!

I can do a lot of great stuff with The Dieters Scale© but I can't go into too much detail here as it takes time.

So instead, we will use a cut down version of it to give you the idea and to put you on the right path.

What we want to do is to find out what type of weight problem you have. To do this we need to put your weight problem into the right Zone on The Dieters Scale©.

Putting your weight problem into the right Zone will help us to see where you are actually living in Fat Land.

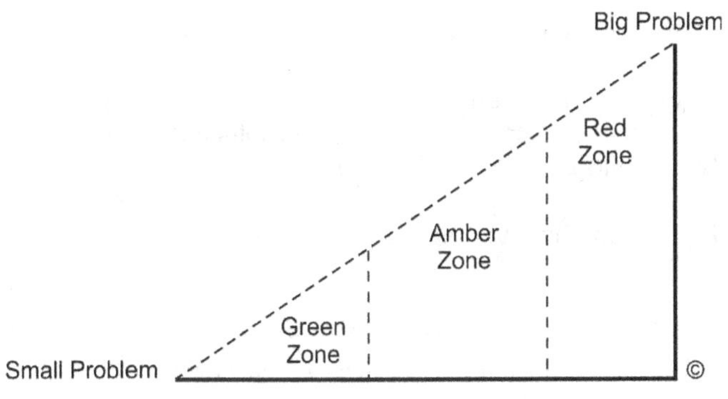

Your weight problem is going to fit into one of the Zones of The Dieters Scale© and we only have 3 Zones:

The Green Zone
The Amber Zone
The Red Zone

Each Zone represents a level of complication and difficulty. So let's have a look at what this means in reality.

The Green Zone is the least complicated and difficult.

The Amber Zone is more difficult and complicated.

The Red Zone is the most difficult and complicated.

So this gives us 3 levels that we can use to begin to see the differences in the weight problems that people with persistent weight problems experience.

Now what you need to understand at this point is that there is no point in cheating. If you cheat you will just fall off one of the Stepping Stones and find yourself back in Fat Land.

In reality you can't cheat this process because you only cheat yourself. And when you are dealing with persistent weight problems and the things that go with weight problems; you can't maintain the results that you achieve by cheating.

If you don't believe me look at your own experiences.

To begin to put you into the right Zone we need to know some simple information which you will have or can easily get. That information is:

1. What is your current weight?
2. What should your weight be?
3. How much weight should you really lose or do you really want to lose?

Now let's use that information.

If you are less than 16lb's (7kg) overweight then you would be in the Green Zone at this time.

If you are more than 16lb's (7kg) overweight but less

than 48lb's (22kg) overweight; then you would be in the Amber Zone.

If you are more than 48lb's (22kg) overweight; then you would be in the Red Zone.

So you see it is quite simple to use The Dieters Scale to begin to understand the level and type of your weight problem.

So which Zone are you in? ________________________

The next thing that we are interested in relates to your dieting pattern.

If you have never dieted before then your experiences with dieting will be different from someone who has done lots of diets or who is always on a diet.

So let's separate out these experiences.

If you have never dieted before or you have only dieted once before; then you will be in the Green Zone.

If you have dieted more than twice but less than 6 times; you will be in the Amber Zone.

If you have dieted more than 6 times or you are always on a diet; then you will be in the Red Zone.

So which Zone are you in? ________________________

The next thing is your ability to stay on a diet.

If you can stay on a diet and lose all the weight that you had planned to lose on that diet; then you will be in the Green Zone.

If you can complete the diet but you can't stick to it and keep it up; then you will be in the Amber Zone.

If you start a diet but can't keep it up and complete it; then you will be in the Red Zone.

So which Zone are you in? ______________________

Our next question relates to your physical appearance, related to your weight and size.

How happy are you with your physical appearance related to your weight and size?

Very happy = Green Zone
Not happy = Amber Zone
Miserable = Red Zone

So which Zone are you in? ______________________

The next question relates to how easy you can move around, do things and how well your clothing fits you.

I find it very easy to move around, to do things and my clothes fit great. = Green Zone

I find it moderately difficult and uncomfortable to move around and do things, and my clothes are uncomfortable. My weight hinders what I do but it does not stop me from doing it. = Amber Zone

I find it quite difficult or impossible to move around and do things because of my weight. My clothing has been replaced by larger baggy items and things like getting in and out of chairs is difficult. My weight stops me from doing things that I would like or need to do. = Red Zone

So which Zone are you in? ______________________

The next question relates to your social life.

Does your weight impact or affect your social life?

No it does not impact my social life in any way. = Green Zone

Yes my weight does affect my social life and it does stop me from doing things which I would like to do. = Amber Zone

Yes my weight has a big impact upon my social life. I have no social life. = Red Zone

So which Zone are you in? ______________________

The next question relates to confidence.

This question has 2 parts.

Part 1.

How does your confidence affect your weight problem?

Not at all = Green Zone
Quite a bit = Amber Zone
A lot = Red Zone

So which Zone are you in? ______________________

Part 2.

How does your weight problem affect your confidence?

Not at all = Green Zone
Quite a bit = Amber Zone
A lot = Red Zone

So which Zone are you in? ______________________

The next question relates to Self-Esteem.

This question has 2 parts.

Part 1.

How does your Self-Esteem affect your weight problem?

Not at all = Green Zone
Quite a bit = Amber Zone
A lot = Red Zone

So which Zone are you in? ______________________

Part 2.

How does your weight problem affect your Self-Esteem?

Not at all = Green Zone
Quite a bit = Amber Zone
A lot = Red Zone

So which Zone are you in? ______________________

The next question relates to Relationships.

This question has 2 parts.

Part 1.

How do your Relationships affect your weight problem?

Not at all = Green Zone
Quite a bit = Amber Zone
A lot = Red Zone

So which Zone are you in? ______________________

Part 2.

How does your weight problem affect your Relationships?

Not at all = Green Zone
Quite a bit = Amber Zone
A lot = Red Zone

So which Zone are you in? ________________________

The next question relates to: How you feel about yourself.

I feel good about Myself all the time. = Green Zone

I feel good about Myself a lot of the time but a fair amount of time I don't. = Amber Zone

I rarely or never feel good about Myself. = Red Zone

So which Zone are you in? ________________________

The next question relates to Control.

Overall when you look at your life and the different things which you do; how "In Control" do you feel?

I am in control of everything that I need to be. = Green Zone.

I am not in control of a number of things that I should be, that I need to be, that I want to be. = Amber Zone.

I hardly control anything, I am totally out of control, and I lost control a long time ago. = Red Zone.

So which Zone are you in? ________________________

The next question relates to exercise.

What we are interested in here is your reality and not what you think you should say. So be honest.

I do actually like to exercise and keep myself fit and I do so on a regular basis. = Green Zone.

I periodically exercise, like when I go on a diet and I think exercise will help me lose weight and look better. = Amber Zone.

I really can't see the point in exercising and I am not interested in it at all. I don't bother. = Red Zone.

So which Zone are you in? ________________________

The next question relates to your Fitness level.

What we are interested in here is your reality and not what you think you should say. So be honest.

I am happy with my fitness level and I can do all the things with my body that I want to do without any problems or difficulties. = Green Zone.

I am not fit and I know that I could be fitter and have a better quality of life if I was. = Amber Zone.

I think that being fit is over rated and I have all these reasons why I cannot get fit and I have a letter from my doctor... = Red Zone.

So which Zone are you in? ________________________

The next question relates to how you actually feel about your weight.

What we are interested in here is your reality and not what you think you should say. So be honest.

I know that I have a problem with my weight and I don't like the fact that I have a weight problem. But I am prepared to do what it takes to deal with this problem now. = Green Zone.

I know that I have a problem with my weight and if I am being honest I have used it as an excuse for different things. If I could take a pill and my weight problem would disappear, then I would. But I realise that it is going to take more than that to fix things and I now accept that I have to do more. = Amber Zone.

Who are you calling fat? = Red Zone.

So which Zone are you in? ___________________________

So now let's total up the answers. This is not a competition and there are not any right or wrong answers. You should have 17 answers.

What we want to get too, is to get an idea of the problem structure that makes up and contributes to your weight problem.

How many Green? ______________________

How many Amber? ______________________

How many Red? ________________________

I would expect that most people will have a mix of answers.

So what does this indicate?

Answers that fall within the Green Zone would tend to fall within what I would call the Normal Zones.

Answers that fall within the Amber Zone would tend to fall within what I would call the Chaotic Zones.

Answers that fall within the Red Zone would tend to fall within what I would call the Dangerous Zones.

Now don't get worried by the names of these different Zones because we are not passing any value judgements here or saying that anyone is in danger.

This is just getting an idea of the shape and difficulty of the problem and how long it may require to improve or resolve it.

About now you might be thinking; how quickly can we fix this thing? So let's answer that and get it out of the way.

The reality tends to be that a Green Zone problem will

tend to be the easiest to work with and the easiest to improve. As a guide this means that these should be quicker to improve than Amber Zone problems.

An Amber Zone problem will be more difficult and tend to take more time and effort than a Green Zone problem.

A Red Zone problem will be the most difficult and will tend to take the most time and effort.

We can't say that it will take (X) months to fix a problem because I don't know what the real problems are and how they may be affected by any other problem. So what we will do is use this guide:

> Green Zone will tend to require the least amount of time to improve or resolve.
>
> Amber Zone problems will take longer than Green Zone.
>
> Red Zone problems will take longer than Amber Zone.

What you need to appreciate is that when it comes to moving out of Fat Land and living in Slim Land, you need to look at the bigger picture.

The approach I like to take is to ask someone; how long they hope to live for?

And the reality is: Do you want to spend a lot of that time in Fat Land or do you want to spend more of that time in Slim Land?

Getting out of Fat Land for a little while is easy! Diet clubs can take you out of Fat Land for a limited amount of time. What they can't do is keep you out!

What we want to do here is to keep you out of Fat Land, move you to Slim Land and help you to build a life in Slim Land. And the truth is that you can't really do this very quickly; it takes time!

Currently you have a Fat Land life and lifestyle; you want to get too and begin living a Slim Land life and lifestyle.

To achieve that result takes time and things have to change and become established into new patterns of behaviour. Rushing things is part of the Fat Land behaviour.

This simple process, with easy to answer questions, can begin to provide us with quite a lot of useful information about the shape and nature of your weight problem.

It also begins to inform us about the journey that you need to take from Fat Land, across the Stepping Stones, and into Slim Land.

Having this information gives you more chances to succeed from the beginning!

One reason why I developed this process was that I could see that too many people were using diets that applied to people who fell into the Green Zone; when they themselves fell into the Amber or Red Zones.

The reality is that if you are someone who falls into the Amber or Red Zones and you use a diet approach suited to someone in the Green Zone; then you are highly likely to fail.

You are trying to put square pegs into round holes!

Making that simple mistake means that your probability of success is going to be low or non-existent.

However; if you use a diet approach suited to the Zones that apply to your weight problem; then your probability of success increases.

> Green level solutions to Green Zone problems.
>
> Amber level solutions to Amber Zone problems.
>
> Red level solutions to Red Zone problems.

Its human nature that most people who diet want quick easy fixes to the problems that they experience. This causes them to make poor choices and to do the wrong things.

If we take the approach of selling everyone a Green Zone dieting solution; regardless of the Zone that they are actually in, then everyone outside of the Green Zone is doomed to failure from the start.

This incompatibility is one of the reasons why diets have an 84% failure rate: Most of the dieters who fail are going to be in the Amber and Red Zones and few will in the Green Zone.

> In reality; it is easier to sell someone the wrong solution which promises fast and easy results; than it is to sell them the right solution which involves more effort and time.
>
> With so many diets the reality is; that the demands of the weight problem that the person has, exceeds the capacity of the dieting solution being applied to it.
>
> It's a case of square pegs and round holes!

In reality few long term weight problems are just about someone's weight.

Their weight often ends up being the visible part of their lifestyle management problems.

Their weight can also be a barometer (indicator) for the level and the difficulty of the other lifestyle problems that the person is dealing with and trying to cope with.

Ongoing weight problems are usually about someone's Lifestyle Management and the different issues and challenges of life that they experience and have to deal with.

With this knowledge you can begin to focus on the right type of preparation for your dieting solution; and this will match with the Zones on The Dieters Scale.

Each Zone will require a different type of preparation because they each need to do a different level of work, over a different amount of time, with different amounts of effort and commitment required.

But don't panic or worry about it because we will start you off with the basic structure that you need to get on to the 1st Stepping Stone and to keep going.

If you fall off the 1st Stepping Stone then see what you missed; or what you forgot; or what you tried to short cut on.

Try not to rush this as it increases your chances of making mistakes and you just won't do what you need to do, in the way that you need to do it.

Remember:

> Falling off a Stepping Stone doesn't mean that you have failed. In this approach: Failure is simply another opportunity to Learn from the Experience and go at it again.

The Dieters Scale©™ & The Human Algorithm® project

The Dieters Scale© is a part of The Human Algorithm® project.

This project is a new way of understanding and working with problems that involve people; in their personal, professional and business lives.

For the purposes of this book, it helps to illustrate that we can look at persistent weight problems in new ways and we can work with persistent weight problems in new ways: More productive and sustainable ways.

We can also work Strategically with simple structures that we can easily understand, rely on and work with.

If we were using The Human Algorithm® to look at a person who had a persistent weight problem; then we would be able to look at their individual problem structure and see how things like their confidence, self-esteem and other issues both effect and are affected by their weight problem.

We would also be able to see where the Strategic points were. These are the points in the problem where small interventions can be made to produce large results for small amounts of effort; or where changes in behaviours at certain points can alter a chain of events and produce a different result.

The Human Algorithm® lets me work with individual people but it also lets me work with problems that affect many thousands and even millions of people; and I can do this in a Strategic way as well.

Persistent Weight Problems are one of the large scale problems that I am working with and I am applying The Human Algorithm® at both the large scale level and at the individual level.

This means that you get a higher level of benefit and a higher level of value from the material in this book and from this approach.

Now you are ready to actually step on to the 1st Stepping Stone.

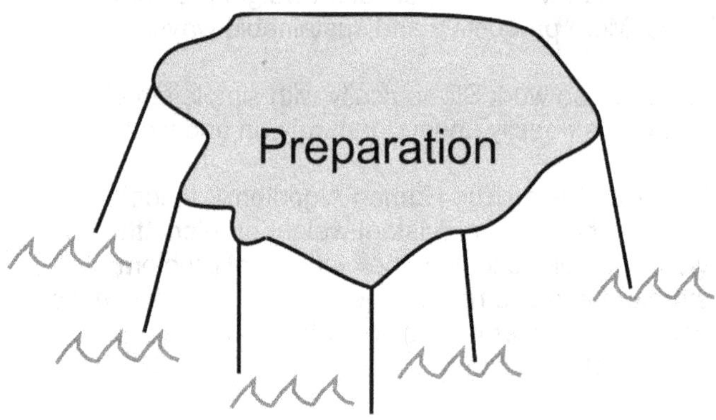

CHAPTER 3

Preparation

Well done for getting this far! You are now ready to actually step onto the 1st Stepping Stone and begin leaving Fat Land behind.

What we do on this Stepping Stone is to prepare ourselves for the 2nd Stepping Stone. The 2nd Stepping Stone is the Diet and Weight Management Stepping Stone.

To be able to get on and be able to stay on the Diet and Weight Management Stepping Stone, we first have to prepare ourselves.

The 1st Stepping Stone is critical and it is usually missed and ignored by 84% of dieters. This part greatly increases your chances of being successful and it creates the foundations for what you will do in the future.

> Warning
>
> If you haven't spent any time considering and answering the questions from the previous chapter; then you need to go back and do so. This will help you to begin to understand that weight problems are different and that they need to be dealt with in different ways.

If you have answered the questions; you will now have an idea of the Zones that you are in on The Dieters Scale©.

Green Zone – Amber Zone – Red Zone

So in our preparation process we need to consider and

prepare according to those Zones.

Most people will have a mixture of Zones and they can consist of Green, Amber and Red Zone. To sort this out is simple.

If you have only Green then do the Green Zone level of preparation. However; even a Green Zone person would be better off preparing more than they think they need too.

So in reality; most people should do the Amber and Red Zone level of preparation. If you do choose to do the Green level of preparation and it doesn't work; then simply move up to the next Zone.

> It doesn't hurt to work as if you are in a level above where you are; it <u>does</u> hurt to work a level below where you are.

This is what is great about this approach: We just have to focus on the right Zone and do the things that are right for that Zone.

Another great thing is that we only need to be able to understand the difference between Red, Amber and Green. Everyone can understand this.

What you have to understand here is that no Zone or colour is bad. What the colour is telling us can be likened to needing to understand the weight of different objects that you are going to have to lift up and move around.

If we had a number of different objects to lift and some were small and some were large; wouldn't we want to know if some were light and some were heavy?

If we know that we are going to lift something light we would take one approach to it. And if we were to lift something large, bulky and heavy; we would take another. It becomes simple common sense that we would apply to the task of lifting things, so that we could do what we needed to do in the right way. Dieting is just the same.

At this point I need to tell you something.

When we are doing the Preparation phase it does not matter if this is your first dieting experience or if you have dieted a hundred times before. Everyone has to prepare. And if you don't prepare in the right way; then you will reduce your chances of being able to reach and stay on the 2nd Stepping Stone. The Diet and Weight Management Stepping Stone!

Put simply; you will be on your way back to Fat Land and have to start over again if you don't do this the right way.

A word of warning here!

Don't put yourself under pressure to succeed the first time. Due to the nature of dieting and weight problems, you need to think of this like playing basketball.

In basketball you will take shots at the basketball hoop but they won't all go in. If you miss one shot you don't stop playing; you keep playing and you get better at it with practice. And this is what many dieters will do with our Stepping Stones Approach; they will keep shooting at their goal and get better with practice.

With this process you work towards your goal by moving through the Zones.

To begin with, a dieter may be deep in the Red Zone. And over time they will move closer to the Amber Zone and move into the Amber Zone.

They may be deep in the Amber Zone and over time

they will move closer to the Green Zone and then move into the Green Zone.

They may be deep in the Green Zone and over time they move into the right part of the Green Zone and achieve what they want.

In each of these cases they get to their goal but not in a simple straight line.

And in reality this is what this whole successful dieting and weight control process is about; getting closer and closer to your goals through a progressive process. This is what you need to always keep in mind and refer back to when things become difficult.

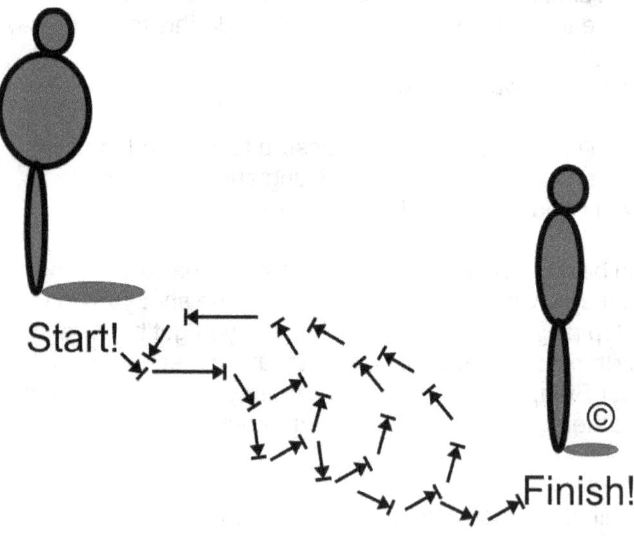

Another way to think of this is to imagine your weight problem being like a train. At the front of the train we have the engine and the engine pulls the different carriages along a set route.

We can add carriages or we can take carriages away and this changes what the train does and how it looks.

Each object on the train represents a part of your weight problem.

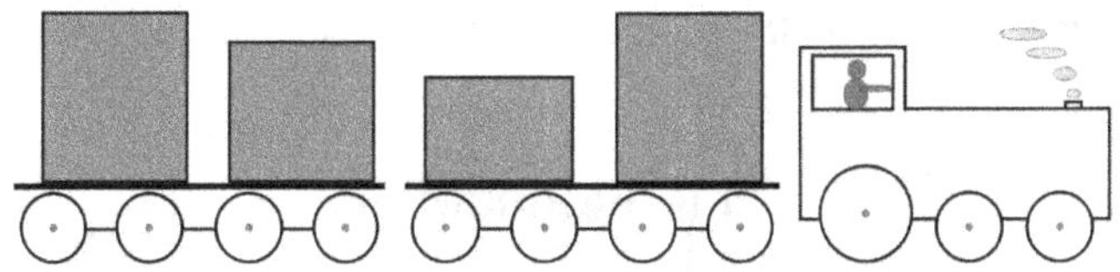

A Green Zone weight problem train.

The carriages (Zones) of your weight problem train are locked together into a structure with a certain size and shape: Your size, your shape, your habits, your lifestyle, your history, etc.

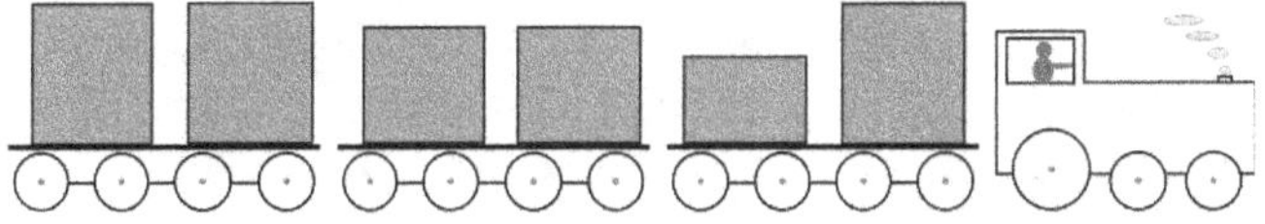

An Amber Zone weight problem train.

If you continue living your life as you are, those carriages on your weight problem train will stay as they are.

However; as you life changes you will add new items to your weight problem train. When you do this your weight problem can become bigger, larger and more difficult to deal with.

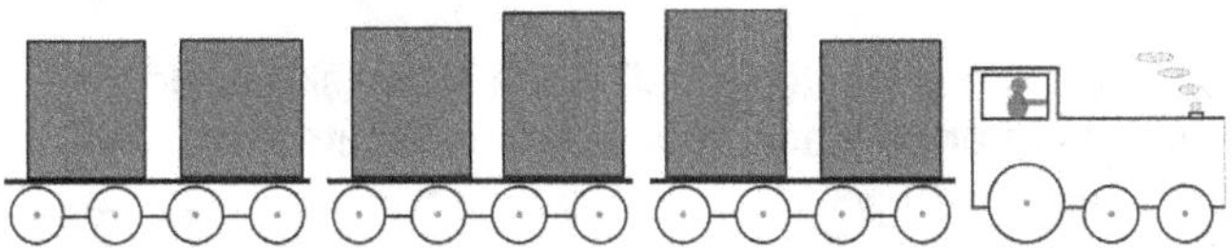

A Red Zone weight problem train.

This is what people who have weight problems tend to do as their weight problem increases and it becomes more difficult to deal with it.

And what we want to do with this approach is to stop you adding new carriages and items to your weight problem train; and begin to change how your weight problem train looks.

Let's get the foundations right!

A truth about weight problems that people don't really talk about is, that in reality: Your weight problem did not just happen overnight.

It wasn't the case that you went to bed one day nice and slim; and then you woke up the following morning with a weight problem.

Your weight problem, and every other weight problem on the planet, evolved over time! It was created a little bit at a time.

And what we are going to do is to use the same processes that you used to create the problem; to undo the problem and create a new structure for you to live with. We are going to work Strategically!

What you need to take from this is something critical.

You have all the skills and abilities required to develop a weight problem. You have proven it to be true because you have a weight problem.

Now we are going to use all those same skills and abilities to undo it and create a different life structure.

So you can't say that you can't do it; because you have already done it once; without realising that you were actually doing it. So you did it instinctively.

However; when you created your weight problem you did not have a plan and you did not prepare for it. Now we are going to plan and prepare to change this. This gives us an advantage.

Preparation with a plan makes it easier!

Now many of you will not get this right the first time. But that is perfectly acceptable and here is why:

> When you were developing your weight problem you made lots and lots and lots of mistakes. But you persevered despite all the mistakes; and you did not let it put you off moving to Fat Land.
>
> You really worked hard at creating this problem over a long period of time. So you have the determination and persistence to create and maintain the problem for a long period of time.

Well now we are going to use what you have already done but in another way – a more productive way!

So what is the preparation that you need to do?

Let's begin with something that no-one has probably told you before. Those of you who are eager to get on with the diet won't like this but it really is something you need to know and understand.

> This makes a huge difference to your dieting experience and the results that you can achieve and maintain.

If you are a Green Zone person and you have had a good or reasonable diet but you have just put on a few extra pounds; then it is probable that your bodies' processes are in the normal functioning range and your body will respond well to a diet programme.

If you are an Amber Zone or Red Zone person then it is probably the case that your bodies are NOT prepared for a diet programme.

This is a critical thing for you to understand as it has a big, big, big impact on your ability to successfully diet and to manage your weight long term.

> MOST PEOPLE WHO ARE IN THE AMBER AND RED ZONES, DIET BEFORE THEY AND THEIR BODIES ARE READY TO DO SO!

The result of ignoring this simple fact is that people who are in the Amber and Red Zones will find it the toughest to achieve the results that they want from dieting.

This is because their bodies, their habits, their lifestyles and all the things which have helped them to live in Fat Land for so long; are still working to keep them in Fat Land.

To change this we need to change the preparedness of their bodies, so that they can use the dieting process in the best way; rather than just messing things up further.

And here's something else you are not going to like:

> Getting your body stable takes about 3 months!

Scream!!!!

But look at this time thing another way. You want to do something different to what you have done in the past; don't you?

By taking time to prepare for a diet we take away all the pressure that you would normally experience when you go on a diet. So we reduce your stress.

And by taking the time to prepare your body and get it

working in a better way, we can increase your chances of getting the result that you want.

So it becomes a win-win process for you; rather than the lose-lose beat yourself up process that you are used too.

The right type of Preparation increases the probability of a successful outcome. And that's what you want; right?

So what is the right type of preparation?

Weight problems that fall into the Amber and Red Zones are too complicated to deal with quickly.

They simply do not respond well to quick simple fixes because they are beyond that. Yeah; you can go on a diet and lose a lot of weight quickly but it doesn't work and you have to deal with all that disappointment again.

We also know that a diet on its own is insufficient to deal with the weight problem; because in reality there is more going on. Yeah I know about all that stuff that you keep secret and that keeps getting in the way of the life that you want to live.

So how do we begin to sort this out?

Earlier I said that the different Zones were like carriages on a train that carried different items. Those different carriages helped to create the shape and size of your weight problem train.

So this means that each carriage and item on your weight problem train is a piece of your weight problem; and to sort out the weight problem train we need to work with the different pieces of it.

What most people try to do is that they try and change the train by working with the engine; rather than the carriages which carry all the freight.

What we are going to do is to work with the train, the carriages, the items and the route that the train normally takes.

Its common sense if you think about it.

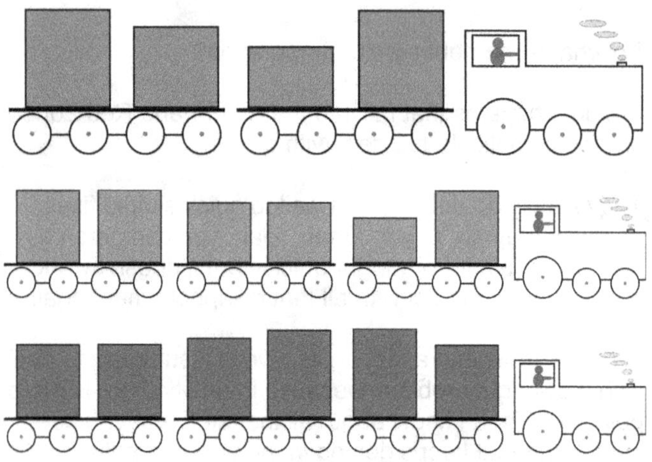

Different dieters have different types of trains, with increasing numbers of carriages and more items being carried along their route.

CHAPTER 4

Focus on the Right Things

What undermines people's efforts and causes so many people who are in the Amber and Red Zones on The Dieters Scale to fail; is this.

> They focus on the diet itself and not on the "weight problem and their lifestyle management that helped to create and maintain their weight problem."
>
> You see; By the time they have moved into the Amber and Red Zones they have more complicated things going on in their lives.
>
> They don't realise that their lifestyle management helped to create and maintain their weight problem and they can't fix their lifestyle management by going on a diet.
>
> In reality; you have developed a Fat Land life and lifestyle; and you want to have a Slim Land life and lifestyle.
>
> To achieve a Slim Land life and lifestyle we need to resolve, improve and manage things in a better way.
>
> So rather than set yourself up for failure; set yourself up for success!
>
> Success is achievable if you do the right things, in the right way, for the right reasons, at the right time.

So let's start doing that.

First we are going to put a Plan together. It will be a Plan that you can keep to and which you can achieve because it will fit your lifestyle and it will fit your capabilities.

Are you up for that?

This Plan can be used by anyone, regardless of whether you are in the Green, Amber or Red Zones and regardless of whether you are male or female, and regardless of your age or any other factor.

MY PLAN TO GET FROM FAT LAND, ACROSS THE STEPPING STONES, AND INTO SLIM LAND. Then you need a plan to stay there.

From Fat to Slim in 3 Steps

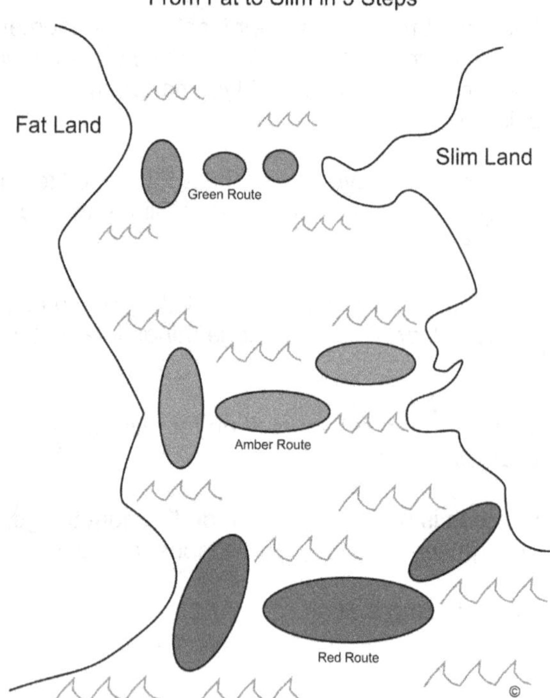

Before we begin there is something that you need to understand.

Every problem, issue and challenge that comes up in your life will be in either a Green Zone, an Amber Zone or a Red Zone.

To deal with these different issues, problems and challenges; we simply take them one at a time. We then progress them forwards to a point where they are stable.

And when one thing is stable enough; then we can work with something else.

We do this in a gradual evenly paced way. No rushing, no panic; make a plan and work with the plan.

We can work with any problem that is affected by your weight and which affects your weight by using the Stepping Stones Approach and following this structure.

- Prepare and practice.
- Act and sort it out.
- Consolidate and put it behind you.

Rushing, putting yourself under pressure and having unrealistic time scales will tend to make you fall off a Stepping Stone.

If you get it wrong and you fall off the Stepping Stone; simply begin the process again from the beginning.

> Take the opportunity to Learn from your mistakes and increase your knowledge and wisdom of yourself and your problems, challenges or issues.

Now we can't do that sort of individual personal work in this book. That type of work is what I can do on the workshops, courses and programmes that I have developed and that I provide as part of The Human Algorithm® Project.

However; we can still achieve successful results; it is just that I cannot personally help you, other than through this book; which is great anyway.

The Stepping Stones Approach is a metaphor; a way of understanding something in another way: An easier way that you can use and refer to, to help you achieve your goals.

What I am trying to get you to understand is that the Stepping Stones Approach will work with any type of persistent weight problem and mixture of other issues; such as confidence and self-esteem. We simply apply the same approach to each one in turn.

Why we are using the different coloured Zones is that we want to match the problem with the right solution for it; and we are using the Zones to help us do this.

> For example; someone whose weight problem falls into the Green Zone will have less of a weight problem than someone whose weight problem falls into the Amber Zone.
>
> If the person who falls into the Amber Zone tries to use the same solution as the person in the Green Zone; then it probably won't work in the same way or at all.

And this goes for all the other problems that we have.

We need to fit the right type of solution to the right type of problem. If we do this then we increase our chances of achieving the result that we want.

We are using The Dieters Scale©™ and the coloured

Zones to help us achieve this.

Keep it simple and don't over complicate it!

Progressing through the Zones

To understand the best way to progress from one Zone to another you simply follow this guide.

If you are in the Red Zone then you want to work towards the Amber Zone.

If you are in the Amber Zone then you want to work towards the Green Zone.

If you are in the Green Zone then you want to work towards the right place in the Green Zone.

This will help you to progress in a steady way and to build up the necessary foundations to move from one place to another and be able to stay there.

Life complicates things for us; the Zones help us to make sense of them and helps us to work with them

Everyone begins their life living in the Green Zone.

As things happen, different parts of our lives move into different Zones.

Over time this creates a complicated mix of different Zones with different levels of problem in each Zone.

As we deal with a problem that is in the Red Zone we don't tend to jump from the Red Zone to the Green Zone.

What we do is we work our way through the Red Zone towards the Amber Zone. Then we move through the Amber Zone into the Green Zone. Then we move to the right place within the Green Zone.

As we make progress in the different Zones, different issues, problems and challenges come up.

However; we can use exactly the same process that we are using in this book to understand and then deal with these.

Once you have used this process and found it useful; then you can continue to use it and apply it to new challenges, problems and issues.

So now let's move on to the Preparation.

Green Zone Preparation

The Green Zone person has less of a job to do and so they will be able to begin a diet sooner. This is because their body should still be within normal ranges, be stable and be able to respond positively to a diet and weight control programme.

If you are a Green Zone person then you probably want to lose the small extra bit of weight that you need to and then keep it off.

If you struggle with keeping the weight off, then my guess would be that the increased weight is as a result of Lifestyle Management issues that are not being properly understood and managed properly.

If this is the case then you really are an Amber or Red Zone person and you should do what they do.

If you are in any doubt about your body's stability then take the time to get your body stable and use that time to prepare to go on a diet. And use that time to look at the other issues, problems and challenges that may be around for you.

In any event it is usually better to over prepare rather than under prepare. If I was in your position I would prepare at the Amber Zone level as the extra preparation would not hurt.

Rather than do separate preparations for all the different Zones I have separated them by a simple method.

The Green Zone person can look at the Amber and Red Zone preparations and take what they need from that and put that into their Plan. This is how we will put the Green Zone Plan together; take what we need from the

Amber and Red Zones.

If you begin to find that quite a lot of their preparation fits you, then move your preparation to Amber and Red Zone levels because this is more likely to be where your problem really fits.

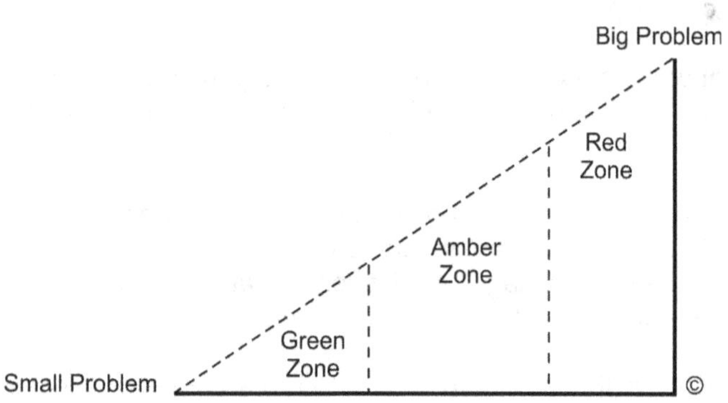

Amber Zone and Red Zone Preparation

Good preparation actually goes further than simply getting things together.

Good dieting and weight management preparation means that while we are preparing, over the next 3 months, to go on our diet; we begin to make things happen which makes getting to and staying on the 2nd Stepping Stone (the diet) easier.

In reality; your body needs to be brought to a condition where it can actually use and benefit from the diet and weight management plan that you are going to use.

First there will be some lifestyle changes that you will need to make before you begin to diet.

The food that you keep around the house can be changed gradually; rather than quickly.

You don't need to tell anyone that you are planning to diet or tell then when you go on a diet, because you are not going to be doing it for their benefit; you are going to be doing it for your own benefit.

You don't need to buy any new clothes or anything like that before you go on a diet. Who needs mementoes of failed diets or the pressure to fit into something that doesn't fit?

You can begin to move about a bit more. Nothing strenuous or over exerting; perhaps just simple walking to help your body work a bit better when you begin to diet?

Don't get mixed up with people who want to be competitive with dieting, weight loss or exercise. You don't need the grief and crap that goes with all that.

See if you can find something, other than food, that makes you feel good about yourself. It might simply be taking some time for yourself each day to walk around the garden or sitting quietly having a hot or cold drink.

Begin to allow yourself some time to consider your life and how you would like to change or improve it in the future. It doesn't have to be big things; often the small things are just as important.

Make a few notes for yourself and keep them somewhere private so that you can look at them from time to time.

Work out how you are going to handle the stress and anxiety from the unexpected problems, issues and challenges that are going to come up as you lose weight and begin to improve your life.

Rather that turn back to food or other behaviour that doesn't help you; how could you manage these things differently?

It is also worthwhile thinking about how you are going to handle things when someone you know wants to put you back in Fat Land or they want to stop you getting out of Fat Land.

It often happens that people who live in Fat Land are easier to control. People who live in Slim Land tend to see the world in more positive ways and are less easy to control. Is this an issue for you?

In my experience quite a lot of people who live in Fat Land are unhappy with their lot in life and when they finally move out of Fat Land and into Slim Land; they change their lives for the better and they work to stay living in Slim Land.

Another thing you might want to consider is this: Who controls what you eat; the person selling you the food or you who gets and pays for the food?

The reality is that you are probably going to have to change something about what you have been eating, when and how much of it you have been eating.

Before you go on any diet it can be a good thing to just practice changing a few things and see how it feels.

If you have got used to eating a lot of take out foods and convenience foods; then your food taste will have been affected by eating this type of food. It makes you like foods that have higher fats, sugars, salt and other ingredients.

When you eat different foods it can take you some time to get used to the taste and textures of them. It can be a good idea to practice with this before you go on any type of diet.

Another thing with food is volume. Large isn't always bad and small isn't always good. It about having some form of balance with volume; and I will use The Dieters Scale and the Red, Amber and Green Zones to help you understand about suitable foods and balancing your diet for living in Slim Land.

Take the time to practice with all of this before you begin any diet proper. That way if things go wrong; well you are not on a diet anyway; you are just practicing!

Anyhow; all of this is just me trying to get you pointing in the right direction. So let's get back to sorting out your weight problem.

CHAPTER 5

Preparation – Part 1 to 5

The pieces of your weight problem that we are interested in at this stage are the following.

1. What are your dieting objectives?

Are you going to lose weight steadily over a period of time in order to get to your "Happy Point" or are you going to do it in stages with a little break in between?

Either way is fine.

If you are going to do this in stages, then at the beginning of each stage you will go over the Stepping Stones from the beginning to the end. You will keep doing this until your final diet, when you will start living in Slim Land.

How much weight do you want to lose with this trip over the Stepping Stones?

If you want to lose a lot of weight quickly then you will fall off the Stepping Stones and find yourself back in Fat Land.

Sustainable weight loss that lets you live in Slim Land does not happen fast for people who are in the Amber and Red Zones. Take your time and enjoy the journey.

2. Who are you relying on to make the trip across the Stepping Stones a success?

In reality; if you need a number of people to co-operate with you, so that you can lose weight; what happens if one or more of them doesn't do what you want?

Your success should really be something that you take responsibility for and you should not make other people responsible for you achieving it. If you want to eat something don't make it someone else responsibility to stop you; accept that that responsibility is yours.

Reliance upon other people is one of the ways that your efforts can be easily undermined and this can cause you to fall off the Stepping Stones.

Don't give other people the power of Fat or Slim over your life; take it and keep it for yourself.

3. Are you really ready to leave Fat Land behind and start living in Slim Land?

Now this might seem like a daft question but the reality is that many people get scared when they really begin to lose weight and get control over their lives.

Part of the reason for this is that problems, challenges and issues that have been hidden in the background and not dealt with; can come back into focus, as your weight recedes as a problem.

When this happens many people do not feel equipped or ready and able to start to sort these other things out. As a result they migrate back to Fat Land and the other problems go out of focus once again.

The result is that they return, unhappily, back to Fat Land, until the next time that they get fed up with living in Fat Land and want to do something about it.

Well the reality is that you don't have to do this!

You can do this journey in stages and take yourself a bit further forwards each time. Then when you really are ready; then you can go over the Stepping Stones for the last time.

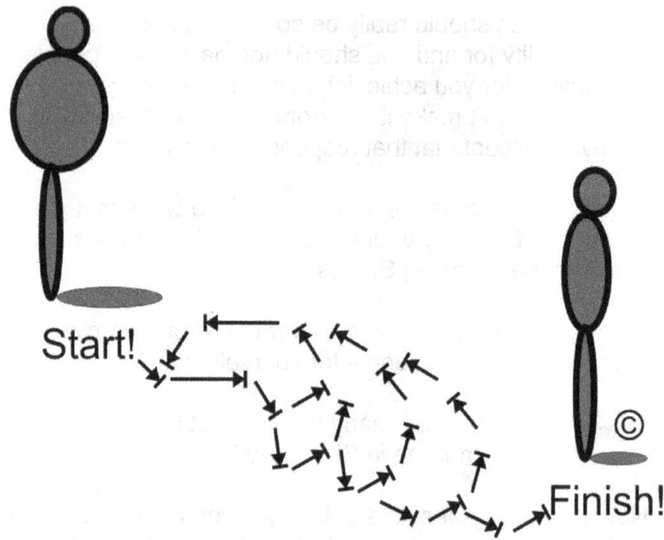

As well as going over the Stepping Stones with your weight, you are also going to go over the Stepping Stones with your other life problems and your lifestyle management issues. These also will be in Zones.

A lot of dieters seem to take the view that they will deal with their weight problem and once that's all dealt with; then they will deal with the other issues.

The truth is that life isn't like that. When these issues come up and they are there; then they need to be looked at. This is life telling you that you can begin the process of improving, resolving or better managing them.

Just like with your diet; you follow the 3 Steps Approach and apply what you are doing with your diet to any other issue, problem or challenge.

You will also apply The Dieters Scale and use the Green, Amber and Red Zones to help you understand the size and complexity of the problem.

I developed this approach to help you to focus on single issues or to combine issues and work with them together.

It really is your choice. If you are not ready you don't have to try and do it all in one go. Take baby steps!

I actually encourage people to take baby steps and to take their time with them. It is much easier to use small bits of effort to move a mountain than to try and move it all in one go.

4. The next point is how are you going to handle the stresses of your life and keep on the Stepping Stones?

Stress is such an easy thing to ignore but it is such a critical piece of the weight problem puzzle.

Stress comes in many different shapes, sizes and forms.

Stress can be created by anything from work, to homelife, to friends, to family, to shopping, to cooking, to sex, to health, to money, to lifestyle, to happiness, to driving, to looking after children, to being overweight, to your diet, to alcohol, to drugs, to not sleeping, to being at home all day, to not getting out and enjoying yourself; and being stuck as a fat person who wants to become slim but who is known for being fat.

The reality is that you have to take responsibility for your own stress and you need to find other ways of handling stress effectively.

The reason for doing this is that your eating habits and patterns will tie into your stress and anxiety management. And for many people the way that they use food will be their stress and anxiety management process.

When you go on a diet, you actually try to remove or greatly reduce the ways that you would normally use food and eating to manage your stress and anxiety on a daily basis.

When you go on a diet you would normally do this without replacing it with something else.

As a result: When your stress and anxiety increases. it has no outlet.

It then bottles up and you increase the pressure on yourself.

As you increase the pressure on yourself, it increases your stress and anxiety until things revert to how they were before; and you once again use food and eating habits to manage your stress and anxiety.

So your stress and anxiety and your use of food and eating habits becomes a circular process which produces negative results for you.

Have a look at the following diagrams.

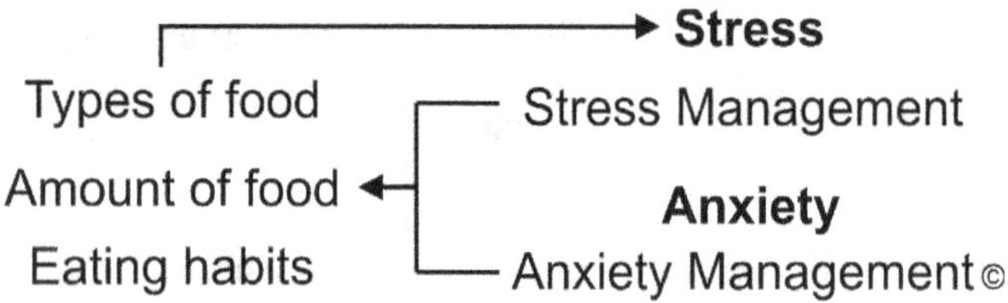

What needs to happen is that we need to change this process and create another process to take its place.

Have a look at the next diagram.

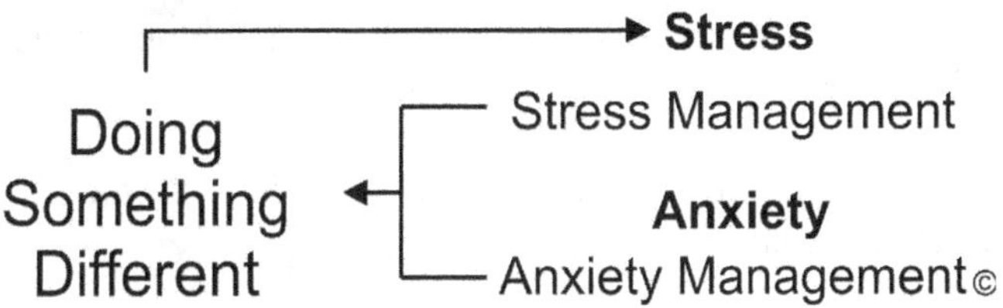

This new process will help you to move away from compulsive and uncontrolled behaviour which affects your eating habits. It will help you to control those urges and to take more control over when you eat, why you eat and what you eat.

Now you don't have to have a single process to deal with everything. The smart thing to do is to have a number of different things that you can do. It might be just taking a break and having a walk, having a coffee, watching a film or programme, having a chat with a friend, etc.

When it comes to stress and anxiety we have to recognise that sometimes it is just plain difficult. But you can make a plan and you can practice different things before you go on your diet proper. If you're not on a diet proper then when you make mistakes and get things wrong it doesn't matter. You can't fail a diet if you are not on a diet.

So you can see that this could be difficult. So imagine how much more difficult this is if you are trying to diet and lose weight; without having an alternative way to managing your stress and anxiety. Its nuts right?

So instead of being stupid; be smart. You are smarter than your weight problem any day of the week.

5. What you need to consider now is the actual diet that you will use.

You want to match the diet to your lifestyle and what you really are willing and able to do.

What you have to understand about any diet where you want to lose weight is this:

> At some point you have to stop losing weight and move on to a process of weight management. This process of weight management needs to be something that you can easily do; so it needs to become an everyday part of your Positive Lifestyle Management.

If you are trying to lose a lot of weight quickly then you probably won't allow enough time for the preparation; as you will want to quickly get to the second Stepping Stone – The diet & Weight Management.

My guess would be that you have done this before and you have been unable to sustain the results or that you failed to achieve the results.

Often I have heard people with weight problems say:

> That this time they would do it quickly and then next time they will do it right.
>
> By the time they get to the next time they say the same thing again. Is this you?

If you read my other book: The Perfect Life Diet For Imperfect People With Weight Problems; you will see a chapter in that book about "The World's Best Diet".

I stand by all that information as you need to tailor any diet that you use to your lifestyle; you can't usually adjust your lifestyle to the diet and keep it up.

This process of adjusting your life to fit the diet is what millions of dieters do every year. This contributes to the very high failure rate of 84%.

> If you have had enough of being a mug then stop behaving like one.

One of the problems that someone in the Amber and Red Zones has is that both their lifestyle management and their dietary practices are out of the normal ranges.

This results in you having chaos and chaotic behaviour in more than one area of your life at the same time.

And what happens when you try to adjust your chaotic lifestyle to a diet. is that you get more chaos. More chaos means more stress and anxiety and then you are in trouble.

So let's take a step back and take another look at the dieting process and look at it Strategically.

There are just 4 things that you need to understand with food and dieting.

1. Nutrition
2. Calories
3. Volume
4. Food flow rate - Frequency

Now you don't need to become an expert on nutrition or

calorie counting or portion control. What you need to understand is the balance between these four components of food and healthier eating; and how you can use these to achieve mastery over any weight problem.

When we get to the 2nd Stepping Stone I will go into the balance between these four components of successful dieting and long term weight control in more detail.

We will be using The Dieters Scale and the Zones to help you understand dieting in a user friendly way that you can use regardless of any diet that you follow.

With The Human Algorithm® Approach it does not matter if you use a diet club, follow a diet plan or make up your own diet. However; there are things which you need to remain aware of and take account off. So let me tell you what these are.

The Human Algorithm® Approach wants you to become independent of any diet or diet plan. You may be part of the 84% of people who normally fail with dieting but the reality is that you can change this.

You can succeed with dieting but any diet can only take you so far on your journey from Fat Land to Slim Land.

A diet can only help with losing weight; it cannot take you to Slim Land and help you to stay there. So this means that any diet club, diet plan or weight control programme has a small window of time where it will be effective for healthy weight loss.

You have to think of this like someone with Depression going to a Doctors and being prescribed Anti-Depressants.

The right way to use medication is that it helps you to feel better so that you are then more able to deal with what is causing and contributing towards the Depression. Medication becomes a tool that allows you to then deal with what is causing the problems.

With a diet club, diet programme and weight control process it is the same. The diet is one of the tools you will use to help you deal with what is causing the problems.

Use the diet to help you get going but don't be seduced into thinking that it will cure all your problems.

In my view, diet clubs and weight control organisations seem to want to sell a lot of other products to dieters.

I personally feel that this is something that you have to be careful about and watch out that you are not seduced by the sales pitches and promises of what you can achieve by using these products.

So what you want to do is sort out what diet plan or programme you are going to use or follow. And understand what it is promising you and what it can really deliver.

Remember that there is an 84% failure rate for a reason.

Marketing promises are easy to make; higher than average results are harder to achieve and maintain. This is what we are after with The Human Algorithm® Approach; higher success rates which become higher long term success rates.

What you have to watch out for are the healthy diets and healthy foods which are not actually as healthy as you are being lead to believe. Just because a company is getting away with making big claims about their products does not make those claims true.

Use your previous experiences with the foods that you know you can and will eat; and use your knowledge of how you manage and control your own lifestyle.

Match what you will and can do now, with the diet or weight management plan that you are going to use. As time goes on you can then change these.

Dave's Diet must have's!

In my view you need to:

1. Eat regular meals.
2. Of regular types.
3. At regular times.

This helps your body to trust that it will have food at regular times, of a certain quality and at regular volumes.

If you lose that regular pattern then your body will adjust accordingly and you will feel the effects.

In my view you should always try to eat a good breakfast and not feel hungry. This helps to stop mid-morning snacking.

You should have a good lunch; if you have snacked and don't feel like eating lunch then what will happen is that you will snack in the afternoon and this will then affect your evening meal.

In the evening you should also have a good meal. This helps to stop snacking during the evening and avoids you then skipping breakfast the following morning.

Now you need to do this even if you don't really feel like it. This is because you need to establish a proper pattern of eating. If you don't then you are introducing chaos into the process; and we know what chaos produces.

CHAPTER 6

Preparation – Part 6 to 10

6. Slowwww down the weight loss and create achievable goals.

If you do the right level of preparation, in the right way; then you will move off the 1st Stepping Stone and you will move to the 2nd Stepping Stone – the diet.

So many people fall of the 2nd Stepping Stone because they rush things. They want things to happen faster and in a linear fashion (just keep losing weight week after week in the same way until they reach their target weight).

The reality is that no-one's body works in that regular fashion; unless they are ill.

Healthy bodies keep adjusting and making use of the resources that they have available to them. Factors like how active you are and the balance of Nutrition, Calories and Volume all come into play.

In my experience; People who want to lose a lot of weight over a short period of time are being seduced by their own desires and ignoring the realities of the life within which they live.

It is much better to take a bit longer to lose that weight than to try and lose it quickly. Fast weight loss is usually followed by fast weight gain and a quick trip back to Fat Land.

7. Dealing with the PLATEAUS.

When you are a few weeks into a diet and you have lost weight what happens?

Your weight stabilises as you hit a plateau; and how do you respond? You cut out more food, increase the amount of exercise that you are doing; and then what happens?

You might begin losing a little more weight. And then what happens? The same thing again – you hit another plateau!

How often can you cut down on your food and increase your exercise before you give up?

Why put yourself through all of that if you don't have too?

What you need to understand is that Plateaus are your body's way of telling you that it needs to adjust. So when you hit a plateau and you change your diet; you prevent your body from adjusting and doing the healthy thing it is trying to do.

So what you are really doing is that you are creating Chaos. And chaos leads to stress and anxiety which leads to...

Plateaus are a real part of being human. As you were putting on weight and moving to Fat Land, you went through different plateaus as you put on weight. You just did not notice them or care about them.

I bet that when you put on weight it did not go on at the rate of 2lb (1kg) per week? I bet that you did not start off slim and then 14 weeks later you were 28lb's overweight?

Of course not!

You can't put weight on like this; and you can't take weight off like this either. This is part of the diet industry nonsense that keeps you in Fat Land.

To be successful; you need to work with your body and not against it.

If you hit a plateau and you have the balance of Nutrition, Calories and Volume right then keep doing what you are doing and wait.

It might take a few weeks or even a few months; but your body will adjust to the point where it can then begin to lose weight once again in a healthy and sustainable way.

This Plateau process is what we are trying to work with during the preparation phase while we are on the 1st Stepping Stone.

We are letting your body settle down and prepare itself for your trip across the Stepping Stones.

Speed is often the enemy of achieving and maintaining good health.

8. Pressure Points! Like holidays and anniversaries.

A weight problem is part of someone's daily life. It lives with them as a companion and as part of their social life.

What we are seeking to do is to help you change those

relationships so that they are more of an asset to you than a burden.

Because of the way that your weight problem and you behave together, we need to consider some of the different situations and circumstances in which you will both find yourselves.

Times, such as anniversaries, holidays and birthdays can become times of great stress and anxiety for someone with a weight problem.

I have come across many people with bitter sweet memories and experiences at such times as these.

What you need to understand is that burying your head in the sand and ignoring your own feelings and emotions is part of what helps to create and maintain a weight problem.

What I hope that you do is that you plan for the holidays, anniversaries and birthdays and think about them beforehand.

As the tension builds leading up to the event your stress is going to increase. How are you really going to deal with it?

Ignoring leads to problems.
Dealing with it leads to solutions!

When you begin to plan for and prepare for difficult times, you begin to take a degree of control. A lack of control is what causes stress and anxiety and we know where that leads.

In reality you need to think of your life as being on an

annual cycle. Each year you will have a birthday and different anniversaries will come and go.

It is the same with holidays. Each year you will hope to have holidays.

If holidays have consisted of eating and drinking as much as you can and putting on lots of weight; then how is the next holiday going to be different?

By planning ahead and being realistic about what you are going to have to deal with; you can change and better manage the results.

9. Preparing your home and other people for your diet and lifestyle management changes.

We live how we are! If you are someone who lives in Fat Land then your home and work space will be that of a Fat Land person.

What we want to do is to prepare for leaving Fat Land behind and for our journey to Slim Land.

Now because we are going to take our time, we can make little changes here and there. As you are not on a diet these are not changes to your diet; they are just preparation.

If you live on your own things can be easier than if you have a family and other people in your household, who also live in Fat Land.

Either way you have a job to do and the better you do it the easier you will find it to get on to the 2nd Stepping Stone and then on to the 3rd Stepping Stone.

So let's see what steps you may need to take with your home and work life.

- De-stress your home and work environment.

At home and at work, you can do simple things which gradually come together and make bigger things.

Simple steps like clearing up clutter, have other people clear up after themselves, clearing away after eating, having a schedule to get household chores done, sharing out the work required in the home, getting outstanding jobs completed, etc.

What you want to get fixed is all that stuff that you have to put up with that you really don't like and that adds to your stress and anxiety.

- Begin managing the food.

If you live on your own or in a household full of other people; you need to begin to manage your food. What this means is that you make simple and little changes by taking baby steps.

If you live in Fat Land then you have a Fat Land diet and that food comes from somewhere. Now what you also have to realise is that many of the foods that help us to put on weight "taste great".

As you move out of Fat Land you don't have to lose great tasting food; but you do need to understand something.

By living in Fat Land you have developed a taste for Fat Land food. Now Fat Land food can be quite different from Slim Land food but it can also be the same as Slim

Land food.

In Slim Land and in Fat Land people lie about foods. In both places people will tell you that their food is healthy and good for you; regardless of whether it is or not.

In both places they will tell you that their food is low fat, low sugar, low salt and so on. People and companies tell lies in their marketing and the promoting of the products that they sell or want to sell.

So don't be seduced by someone who is telling you that they sell food to people in Slim Land and you should buy it. Later on I will give you a guide to understanding the foods that you need and you can apply this to help you.

So what you need to manage are things like treats. Do you really need that emergency supply of comfort food that you keep? If it is easily accessible then it is easy to eat on impulse.

Look at your normal daily diet. How many take-outs are you having each week? Look at any food the morning after and see if you would really eat that stuff cold?

Look at convenience foods. Are you buying prepared meals and then just heating them up?

Look at those drinks that you have through the week. How many fizzy drinks are you having? Are you drinking wine? Do you have too much sugar with your hot drinks?

As you look at these different things there will be things that you can easily change and improve. Now is the time to begin to do this because you are not on a diet and there is no pressure to get it right. You have the time to experiment.

Now something else that you need to understand is that you may have developed “the taste” for Fat Land foods because they often have extra fats, sugars and other additives that our bodies get used to quite quickly.

As a result it will take time to lose the taste for Fat Land foods. These are the ones that have the extra hidden sugars, fats and other things that can get you into trouble.

Now something else that you need to understand is that the same food does exist in both Fat Land and in Slim Land. Let’s use pasta as an example.

Slim Land pasta will be cooked in the same way as Fat Land pasta. It is what is added to it as it is cooked and after it is cooked that alters things.

Fat Land pasta may have a very tasty highly flavoured sauce mixed in with it. It needs to be highly flavoured because Fat Land pasta eaters have got used to highly flavoured foods. To achieve the high flavour, additives and other ingredients will have been added into the sauce. It won’t be the pasta that is the problem; it’s the sauce.

Slim Land pasta will also have a sauce added to it that is very tasty. But a Fat Land person has got used to a sauce that is full of other ingredients and it does not have the same punch. By comparison it can taste bland.

So you need to allow the time for your taste to change and be able to appreciate more subtle taste and flavours.

As you are not on a diet; this is a good time to experiment with that.

- Prepare other people.

When I have worked with people to help them move from Fat Land to Slim Land, we often end up encountering a problem with other people.

These can be friends, family, work colleagues or just people that you know and come into contact with.

What you need to understand and appreciate is that all these people have got used to you living in Fat Land, having a Fat Land lifestyle and looking as if you belong in Fat Land.

Now you are going to change how they perceive you and how they have got used to thinking about you and treating you.

In effect: They will have to adjust with you as you move across the Stepping Stones from Fat Land to Slim Land and begin living in Slim Land.

And like all adjustments; they don't always go smoothly.

You need to prepare yourself that other people may let you down. They may put you under pressure to go back to Fat Land and behave like the person they are used too.

You need to be prepared for this and for those closest to you to do the unexpected; when you least expect it and when you are least prepared for it.

I tell you this because this often happens and these can be very short and quick ways for you to end up back in Fat Land.

So start to make the little adjustments that you need to make. Drop little hints that you are going to make some small changes. Then begin making those small adjustments and changes. When you do so; keep to them!

This way is less stressful and more easily achievable.

10. Putting some of the changes in place before the diet proper.

It is a good idea to begin putting some of the changes in place before you consider starting your diet proper. It allows you and other people the opportunity to get used to those changes without any of the pressures of the real diet being there.

You will also need to begin practicing with your new ways of managing and dealing with the stress that you will experience and the stressful and anxious situations that you will find yourself in.

Get used to the stress and anxiety management and begin using it. Then when it comes to the diet proper you will be familiar with your new ways of handling and managing stress and anxiety.

What you need to remember is that you are on the 1st Stepping Stone. If things go wrong and you fall off; simply go back over the process and start again. If you can't stay on the 1st Stepping Stone then how will you stay on the 2nd and the 3rd?

This isn't a race. This is the rest of your life and we want you to live for a very long time; being happy and having a great life.

CHAPTER 7

Preparation – Part 11 to 15

11. Getting used to the Stress Management before the diet proper.

Once you have your new stress and anxiety management strategies in place you can begin practicing them and trying them out.

You know what types of situations make you nervous and anxious; and you know what you normally do during and after those situations. So why not take an easy one of these situations and see what happens in that situation when you apply your new ways of handling stress and anxiety.

Practice will help you when you do go on the diet proper. It will make you familiar with the feelings and emotions that you are going to experience during and after the event.

With some things you may have to practice more than others. The reason for practicing is that in different situations you will have:

- Muscle memory
- Emotional memory
- Psychological memory
- Social memory

And each one of these will be using your Fat Land

responses; the ones that you have learned and been using all the time that you have been living in Fat Land.

You need the chance to introduce new responses that can help you move out of Fat Land and this gives you the chance to practice with them before you begin any diet.

12. Eating regularly and working with 3 meals a day to prepare your body.

Your body needs regular amounts of food, at regular times. This helps to produce a stability with your food intake that your mind and body can rely upon.

Go back to number 5 and read the Diet Must Haves again. This simple process of eating regularly and predictably is what will help your body to stabilise and be ready to lose weight when you go on that diet.

By starting the process at this stage you can get used to it first and correct any problems before you go on any diet proper. If you wait to do this until you go on that diet proper then you will increase your chances of falling off a Stepping Stone.

Remember; if you are an Amber or Red Zone dieter then it can easily take 3 months or more before your body will achieve stability and be able to properly respond to a diet.

You can use that time to practice and get these things in place.

13. Getting your food stash out of harm's way.

If we were dealing with alcohol addiction we would want

to put distance between an alcoholic and alcohol. If we were dealing with a drug addict we would want to put distance between the drug addict and their drugs of choice.

When the alcoholic or the drug addict is in a stressful, anxious or difficult situation, their proximity to their drug of choice determines how easy it is for them to get it and then use it.

And in reality; comfort food, reward food, compensation food, stress food, anxiety food, boredom food; are the same type of thing.

Your proximity to those foods, of your choice, when you are stressed or anxious determines how easy it will be for you to consume them.

What happens at those times is important because you are re-enforcing your old habits and making sure that you continue to live in Fat Land.

Many people who live in Fat Land will have stashes of food that they will use in emergency situations. If that stash is easy to get to, then you will find it easy to eat it.

How will you manage to change if it is too easy to get to your food stash?

14. Moving your body about before eating.

Over recent years there have been medical studies looking at how our bodies process and manage food.

Some of these have focused on the way that our bodies handle and manage food in situations where someone has been moving around prior to eating and where the same person has not been moving around prior to eating.

These Studies have shown that our bodies handle food better and in healthier ways if some form of mobility has occurred before the consumption of the food.

What this means for the dieter is that a few minutes of simple exercise, such as a short walk, can help your body to better manage and process the food that you are about to eat.

This becomes a useful thing to know because at times you may find that you are going to go out for a meal or going to eat with friends and you don't want to miss the event. So being mobile shortly before you eat could help your body to manage and process the food better.

Like everything this needs to be done with moderation.

15. Walking your way to Slim Land.

If you are an Amber or Red Zone dieter then you may not be as fit as you should be. Now being fit is often misunderstood by people with weight problems. Being fit doesn't mean that you need to become an athlete.

Being fit is about the level of health that you need to have to enjoy and maintain the lifestyle and quality of life that you want to have and enjoy.

So if you want to be someone who lives in Fat Land and you don't mind that you can't walk anywhere, or that you can't run, or that you can't do activities that require you to do anything physical or that you easily get out of breath and that you have no muscle tone; then fine.

If you do mind any of that and you want to improve and change your life; then what can you do?

Well I am an advocate of walking. Just plain old simple walking that does not require any fancy gear or products.

In my book: The Perfect Life Diet For Imperfect People with Weight Problems; I look at things like walking and how to use this simple activity to help you get and maintain the necessary level of fitness for your lifestyle.

In reality; if you can walk, then you can begin the process of getting fit. Walking can also be a good way of dealing with stress, anxiety and boredom.

Why not give it a try before you go on the diet and see what happens?

CHAPTER 8

Preparation – Part 16 to 20

16. Dealing with all the media pressures.

This might seem like an odd thing for me to say. You're unlikely to be a celebrity and have the press trying to take pictures of you. (If you are a celebrity and you are reading my book; why not give me an endorsement?).

Anyway: What I am talking about is all the background media pressure that most people come into contact with every day but may not notice: The magazines, the television, films, the Internet and the radio.

When you have a weight problem you tend to be constantly looking at other people and how they look, what they are wearing and is there any fat showing.

The reality is that when we get over the age of 30 we don't have perfect bodies. Life takes a toll of all of us and we have to do work to keep in shape and look good.

Any image that you will see in the media can and probably has been computer enhanced. This means that someone will have imperfections removed, legs can be made longer, bodies can be made thinner, skin can be made perfect, hair can be made to look fantastic and so on.

When you see an image in the media and you try to conform to this; you may as well try to conform to a dolphin. You see you are trying to conform to something that is not real, not sustainable and a fictitious creation of the media.

The reality is that just about everything that you will buy, want or need is going to be subject to marketing spin.

Marketing spin is used because they usually need to provide you with an aspiration to buy into, in order to sell to you.

Take back your life from the media and work out what you really want to be and then go for it. They need you more than you need them.

17. Don't buy any new clothes.

I have a Mother, 2 sisters, lots of Aunts and cousins. The number of times that I have heard people say that they have bought new clothes to get into when they lose weight.

My advice is: Don't do it!

For most people it becomes another pressure and if they fail on the diet it becomes a permanent reminder of that failure. Haven't you had enough crap in your life!

Why not treat yourself when you have achieved a stage of success.

If you are losing weight in stages, then when you hit a significant stage and your weight and lifestyle are stable; then treat yourself to something.

In the preparation stage, which is where you are now, you can have a plan to treat yourself to something at a later stage in the process; but wait until you get there and you know that you are going to stay there before you celebrate.

Don't distract yourself by buying what you can't use now.

18. Tough choices and tough decisions.

We can't avoid them. We all have them and we all have to make them. Tough choices and decisions are going to have to be made and stuck too.

If you are going to move from Fat Land to Slim Land then it is likely that you are going to have to make these tough choices and tough decisions at some point along this journey.

In reality the best way to do these things is to see them coming and to prepare for them.

If you look at your life, you will have an idea of what you are not happy with and what you will need to deal with at some point. Well eventually some point arrives and you either back off from it and try to leave it or you get in there and deal with it.

If there are major issues that you will need to deal with and you cannot deal with them on your own; try and get the right sort of help.

I find that sitting down and writing out the problem helps me. I also write out the preferred solution and then see what process I need to go through to get the result that I want.

At times that old saying: You can't make an omelette without breaking eggs comes to mind.

What this really means is that you can't leave everything as it is and change it at the same time. I have noticed that quite a lot of people try to do this.

These things can be challenging but if you adopt the Positive Lifestyle Management Approach that I advocate; then you can begin to live a positive life and seek to change your life in positive ways.

What this is about is how you get to Slim Land and how you will continue to be able to live in Slim Land and have a great life.

Issues that cause problems in your life and which remain unaddressed are ones that can shorten your stay in Slim Land and carry you back to Fat Land.

Develop ways of better managing and dealing with problems, issues and challenges that you will face in life.

19. Snacks!

Snacks can be great but let's face it there is a lot of crap things wrapped up to look nice that people want us to buy.

When it comes to snacks, and all the food and drink that you are going to consume, what you need to understand is this:

> Lots of people put water with crap and call it gravy!
>
> Just because it is for sale; it doesn't mean that it is good for you; or that it has had all sorts of test to make sure that it is safe to go on the market; or that it is safe for you to eat lots of them.

In reality if you are eating lots of snacks then there is something wrong with your diet. If you are eating 3 meals a day then you have to look at why you are snacking.

Are you using snacks to manage stress, anxiety or boredom?

I am not saying don't snack but I am saying that it has to fit with your journey from Fat Land to Slim Land and your being able to live in Slim Land.

This means altering your Fat Land snacking habits and changing them to Slim Land snacking habits.

20. Alcohol, drugs and medication.

In your life, with your diet and your lifestyle management, you have to look at what you are doing and why you are doing it.

If you are consuming a lot of alcohol then this will be having a number of different effects and affects upon you.

These will be physical and psychological and it will also affect your weight and how your body processes and manages food.

In my view it is better if you consume no alcohol or very little alcohol. One of my reasons is that although alcohol can be fun and pleasant; it is in reality a poison for human tissue.

It is a poison that we can tolerate and use and achieve different results from; but it is still a poison and it will kill and harm people when used in large quantities.

Alcohol also alters our moods and perceptions. This is one reason why so many people use alcohol at times of stress and anxiety. They also use it to relax and let themselves go at parties.

From the point of view of someone living in Fat Land; alcohol also has lots of calories. Drinking too much alcohol makes you put on weight.

If we apply The Dieters Scale to alcohol, then no alcohol is the Green Zone.

As you consume alcohol you move out of the Green Zone and into the Amber Zone. As your consumption of alcohol increases above 20 units per week, you move out of the Amber Zone and into the Red Zone.

I have seen an increasing number of women whose alcohol consumption falls into the Red Zone.

So this provides you with a simple way of understanding the effects and affects of alcohol.

When it comes to drugs and medication we need to segment these. Are they elective (you choose to take them) or are they are prescribed (you have a genuine medical reason to take them).

Now there are very valid reasons for people to take prescription medication. There are also people who abuse prescription medications.

With the elective use of prescribed and none prescribed drugs, you have to ask why you are doing so. Is it to make life more bearable?

Are you using it to help you cope with something?

What you need to consider is how the inappropriate use of alcohol, drugs and medication will fit into your new life in Slim Land and your desire to continue to live there.

Is it better to begin to address these issues before you go on a diet?

Only you can really answer this question.

CHAPTER 9

Preparation – Part 21 to 30

21. Eating out.

No-one likes to be a party pooper!

At one time or another you are going to be in a situation of eating out. The question then becomes one of:

Are you going to eat out or are you going for a blow out?

Enjoying eating out is different from stuffing as much food into you as you can stand. One is fun and the other has a good chance of making you ill.

You know I am not the fat police. And in reality you don't need the fat police. If you think that consuming as much food as you possibly can, as often as you can is fun; who am I to get in the way of your fun.

All you need to do is take the responsibility for all that fun that you are having. Simple!

Enjoying a meal out is something that everyone can do. Doing it too often will present you with a challenge that you are going to have to deal with.

The challenge is that you lose control over what goes into the food that you eat; and it is usual for restaurants to use more fats, sugars and other ingredients to increase the flavours and taste of their food.

And let's face it: you have a problem with food and that is why you are in Fat Land.

Eating out and enjoying it is part of your positive lifestyle management. While you are at this preparation stage it could be very useful for you to begin managing eating out in a positive and productive way.

Remember: Go for a meal out; not for a blow out!

22. Holidays.

Holidays can be great fun and a real break from the difficulties and challenges of everyday life. They are also events where so many dieters get into trouble.

Real life continues all the time; even on holidays.

The body that you had before you went on holiday; is the same one that you have on holiday; and it will be the same one that you have after the holiday. So why would you treat it any different?

The truth is that going on holiday is about fun, relaxing and having a good time. So enjoy yourself!

What you do have to remember is that your body still has the same rules on holiday as it has the rest of the time. So if you are in the process of stabilising your weight and you go on holiday; then stick with the 3 meals a day process.

At any time you can really enjoy your food. You just have to watch the blow outs and the Fat Land diet.

You don't have to deprive yourself of anything but you will have to watch your volume of consumption.

Consume (eat and drink) too much and you can undo a lot of good work in the course of a couple of weeks.

Especially if you are trying to get your body stable.

If you do mess things up then you need to go back and start over again. The 3 month period will begin again.

Is it worth throwing everything away that you are working towards?

Will you do that every time that you go on holiday somewhere?

The reality is that if you do: Then you are really living in Fat Land and just visiting Slim Land from time to time.

23. Christmas and other festivals.

Every year there is going to be festive holidays and feast days. Fantastic!

Enjoy them and have fun.

Use the information from these different sections and work out a plan so that you can enjoy and get the most out of the festive break and feast days.

Remember that a feast is not a blow out. A feast is a celebration and celebrations are about enjoyment.

Feasts are not about being so stuffed that you cannot move.

Just remember what you are working towards and how easily you can throw away all that good work if you act like a Fat Land resident who has no self control and no self respect. You are better than that and you are worth a whole lot more than some idiot who lets food rule them; rather than serve them.

Become the master of your own body and what you want to do with it and what you want to put in it. Remember that once it is in your mouth you lose control over it.

24. Treats.

Oh; don't you just love treats. I know that I do!

And once again you have to understand what a treat is and why you are having it.

Does the treat need to be food? In reality; as you begin to move out of Fat Land and develop your lifestyle management, you will find that other things can be treats; other than food.

A nice day out at the beach. Watching a good film. Having a BBQ (yes it involves food but you can manage it right!). Going for a walk somewhere nice. Having some "Me" time. These are just some simple examples of what a treat can be.

Having a treat that involves food is OK. What you have to understand is that just because we call it a treat, that the rules that govern our bodies are still there. If we eat a load of fast food until we are completely stuffed; it is still fast food that we have stuffed ourselves with.

If we eat lots of chocolate; it's still chocolate. If we drink lots of alcohol; it's still alcohol.

The real secret of a treat is that we enjoy the treat until we have had enough of it.

If we have the treat too often then it stops being a treat and it becomes normal and every day. By its nature a treat is something that we do occasionally.

So enjoy the occasional treat that involves food but remember these simple guidelines.

25. Tough days!

As we all live real lives there are going to be tough days.

Very few people avoid having tough days. So if we know that they are going to happen; plan for them.

At the moment if there is a tough day what do you do?

Does it involve food?

In the future you don't want to revert to using food as a means of managing your stress and anxiety. You want to use other ways of doing this.

On bad days you will use these other ways to manage and handle the stress and anxiety. If they are insufficient then you will need to work on some more and learn some new things.

What you need to understand about stress and anxiety management is that you don't stop feeling and experiencing stress and anxiety; the purpose is that it helps you to manage and control how it affects you and how you respond to it.

It's like soldiers and fear. Soldiers do feel fear and they have to learn how to live with it and manage it. If they let the fear take over it creates problems and they can't do their jobs.

26. Catastrophes.

No-one likes it when something bad or something really bad happens.

The truth is that the really bad things in life don't tend to happen that often but they do happen.

When really bad things do happen it is important not to become self-destructive. Hurting yourself does not help the situation.

In bad situations my view would be to do that which needs to be done.

It is usually better to assess the situation and understand what you are really dealing with; and then to work out a plan for how to manage and deal with things.

In all cases life goes on and those of us who survive have to continue to live. The best testament that survivors of catastrophes can make is to survive and live their lives to the best of their abilities.

27. Booze.

Haven't we already done alcohol? Yes we have but now I am going to talk about booze.

Why booze? In recent years more and more women have become big drinkers of wine and other alcoholic drinks.

Many women can easily drink a bottle of wine a day and certainly several bottles a week. Many will also drink lots of beer and spirits such as Vodka.

Why are we calling it boozing? It's because of volume, frequency, and why?

It's how much they are drinking, why they are doing so and how often they are doing so.

Boozing is using alcohol in the same way that someone uses food; in the wrong ways.

Boozing gives you the opportunity to take on thousands of calories, to hurt your body and mind; and to make yourself ill.

Boozing is another form of stress relief, anxiety management, making yourself feel better (temporarily) and being one of the lads or one of the girls.

Boozing is a blunt way of dealing with things by anesthetising yourself with lots of alcohol.

Boozing takes a toll of the body regardless of whether you are male or female.

Boozing may involve binge drinking or consistent and regular drinking.

Boozing helps you to take on lots of Calories quickly. Someone drinking in the Red Zone can easily take on several thousand booze related Calories each week or each month.

Go back to number 20 and read that again.

28. Food Addiction

In my book: The Perfect Life Diet For Imperfect People With Weight Problems; I spend some time looking at food addiction and whether it is something that I consider to be real. If you think you may be addicted to food then you should read this book.

29. Weighing Yourself

How often are you weighing yourself and why are you

doing so?

If something is going to help keep you in Fat Land; it is going to be the weighing scales.

Weighing and measuring yourself on a regular or frequent basis can mean that you end up feeling good or bad according to what weight the needle points at.

Weighing scales are more important if you are underweight; rather than overweight. This is because someone underweight has more risk to their health than someone who is overweight. This is because their bodies may simply not have enough nourishment and nutrition to keep them alive.

When people are overweight it is a different type of problem.

If you are overweight then weighting yourself something like once a month is best. And when you do weigh yourself the result needs to be considered along with a number of other factors.

Your body will vary by a couple of pounds according to what you have eaten and drank and when you did so.

Your body can also vary by a couple of pounds according to how well your digestive system is working and what is going through your digestive system.

Your body can also vary, especially in women, according to things like your menstrual cycle.

So with just these three things we could have 5-6lbs (3kg) of weight variation.

What we are really interested in is your journey from Fat Land to Slim Land. And on that journey I <u>don't</u> need you to weight yourself because there can be many positive things which are happening which can make you seem as if you are getting heavier; when in reality it is your body working better.

Positive things that can happen, which can make it look like you are putting on weight include: putting on more muscle.

In this process we need to look at your weight when you begin and we need to look at your weight when you are in Slim Land and comfortable with your weight. This will provide your Happy Point: The point at which you are happy with your weight.

The diet industry normally wants you to keep looking at that scale and to continue being influenced by what it says.

Why listen to an industry with an 84% failure rate!

I don't need you to keep weighing and measuring yourself as it gives you the wrong messages and it keeps you fixed in Fat Land.

I am more interested in where your real "Happy Point" is.

30. Prepare yourself

Now that you are seeing and understanding what proper preparation consists off, the next thing is to prepare yourself for actually taking action.

Please don't be put off by preparation because you don't have to do it all in one go. It is not a race!

Preparation is about bringing the things together that you need to do a job. In this case it is the job of getting from Fat Land to Slim Land and then living in Slim Land.

When you are successful with that, it will be something that you will want to do for the rest of your life. So this is something for the long term.

If you take the time that I am suggesting and you begin to put these things in place and begin to practice using and doing them; then you will find that by that process you are preparing yourself to take action; and you are practicing the things which you need to practice; before you begin the diet proper.

You will be doing what is necessary to stay on the 1st Stepping Stone and to enable you to get on and stay on the 2nd Stepping Stone.

Common parts of a weight problem include the following.

Now I am not saying that your weight problem has been affected by these; or that these have affected your weight problem; because I don't know you. But have a think about it. Does any of it feel right to you?

Your Pattern of eating – When you eat, what you eat, why you eat.

How Much you eat.

What Triggers your eating.

Are you eating 3 times a day in a regular and predictable pattern or is it irregular.

Do you have food with you or easily accessible to you a lot of the time or all of the time.

Are you eating comfort foods a lot.

Are you eating processed foods a lot.

Are you snacking a lot.

Are you missing regular meals because you snack too much.

Do you really know what sensible eating habits really are.

Does eating make you feel safe, make you feel in control, provide you with a focus.

Have you got into the habit of eating junk food.

Have you got into the habit of wanting and eating fast

food all or most of the time.

Do you feel out of control.

Do you understand what a healthy diet is by comparison to an unhealthy diet.

Would you like to have a healthy diet rather than an unhealthy diet.

Would you like to ease into a healthier diet that supports you living in Slim Land.

Has your lifestyle changed to support you living in Fat Land.

Are you physically healthy.

Are you fit enough.

What are your relationships like.

What is your confidence like.

What is your self esteem like.

Do you get enough “Me” time.

Is your life chaotic.

Are parts of your life out of control.

How do you manage stress.

Do you know what stress is.

Do you need to learn how to manage stress better.

Do you need to learn how to be more assertive.

Do you understand the difference between aggressive and assertive.

Do you get angry with yourself.

Do you get angry with other people.

How do you control and manage your anger.

How do you control and manage other people's anger.

What legacy issues are affecting your quality of life.

What direction do you want your life to take in the future.

Do you need help achieving direction and purpose for your life.

A simple thing to understand is this:

> Just about everyone is capable of moving from Fat Land to Slim Land and staying there.
>
> Many of you will need to take the Stepping Stones Approach more than once. Each time you will learn and progress forwards but eventually you will reach Slim Land and be able to stay there.
>
> It doesn't actually matter what type of weight problem you have. It doesn't matter what level and number of associated issues that you have.
>
> Any weight problem and its associated issues can be resolved, improved or better managed so that someone can reach their "happy point".
>
> Have faith.

Chapter 10

In Summary

Amber and Red Zone dieters need to allow about 3 months or more for their bodies to achieve stability.

If you diet before your body is stable then all you are doing is adding to the problem. You may lose weight but I don't think you will achieve and maintain the weight that you want.

Achieving stability means that you will need to prepare for your diet by eating 3 meals a day: Regular meals, regular amounts, and regular times. This helps to balance the Food Flow Rate that your body needs.

In preparation for going on a diet you need to begin managing your food.

Look for problems that will affect your ability to diet and see how you can manage them better before you begin any diet.

Prepare your home and your workplace by making small changes and reducing problems.

Before your diet proper; start practicing with ways of managing stress and anxiety that does not involve using food.

Try out different foods to see whether or not you will be able to use them and keep them in your diet long term.

Look for "hot spots" in the coming year such as holidays, anniversaries, family visits, etc. Things that can cause you problems, issues and challenges that can effect your diet.

Write down your dieting goals. Test them out. Are they really what you want?

How much pressure are your dieting goals going to put you under?

Work out what diet you are going to use. Is it one of your own, someone else's or are you going to use a diet club?

Can your diet change from being a weight loss diet to being a weight management process that you can easily incorporate into your daily life? It needs to be able to do this or you need to be able to transition from the diet to a weight management process that fits how you want to live.

Should you lose a bit of weight and practice all this stuff before you go on a diet? This can take the pressure off of you and let you practice and make mistakes at a time when you are not dieting.

What are the other problems, issues or challenges that are part of your weight problem?

Do you understand where these fit within The Dieters Zones? Are they Red Zone issues, Amber Zone issues or Green Zone issues?

Looking at these different things; are there any that really should be addressed or managed a bit better before you begin your diet?

If you follow this process what you will be doing is dealing with your weight problem at different levels.

Part of the preparation work and practice that you do now will begin to benefit you when you move on to the 2nd Stepping Stone; the diet and Weight Control

Stepping Stone.

Part of the preparation work and practice that we are doing now will benefit you when you move on to the 3rd Stepping Stone; Positive Lifestyle Management.

And part of the preparation work and practice that you do now will benefit you when you get to Slim Land and it will help you to live in Slim Land.

At each Stepping Stone there needs to have been preparation work and practice in order to make it easier for you to stay on the Stepping Stone; but also so that you can achieve the things that you need to achieve in order to progress to the next stage.

If you have done the preparation and practice that you need to do; then you can move on to the next Stepping Stone.

Always remember:

> If you make a mistake or get things wrong; that each mistake and error is an opportunity to learn and get it right next time.
>
> Each failure is an opportunity for knowledge and wisdom about what you need to do to be successful.

On each Stepping Stone you will be preparing, practicing, and using what you have previously prepared; and you will be adjusting whatever needs to be adjusted.

It is just like a sailing ship which has to keep correcting its course so that it can reach its destination; you will become like the sailing ship and correct and adjust to reach your goal.

The 2nd Stepping Stone

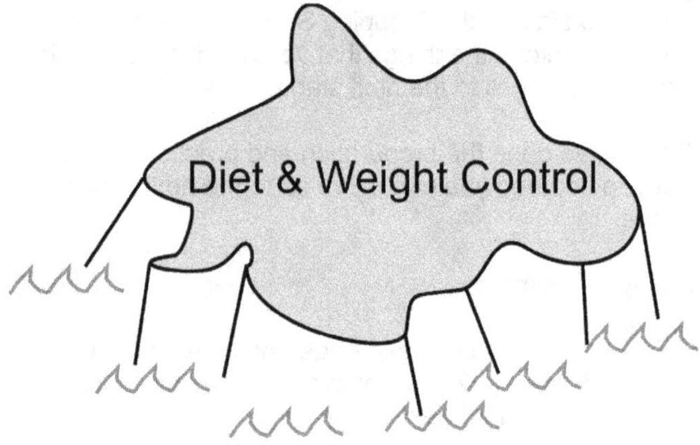

When choosing your diet or Weight Management process you should take a note of the following:

> Any diet or Weight Management process has to be able to fit into your lifestyle.
>
> As your lifestyle changes from a Fat Land lifestyle to a Slim Land lifestyle; your diet or weight management process has to be able to do so as well.
>
> A quick weight loss diet or fad diet lacks the structure that you need to maintain the results.

Chapter 11

How to succeed on the 2nd Stepping Stone

The 2nd Stepping Stone is where most dieters try to start from and it is where most of them actually fail. For most of them it is not their fault, as they have been lead to believe that what they are doing is the right thing to do.

Now, I hope, you know better!

I am trying to help you to equip yourself with the tools and knowledge that you will need to be successful on the 2nd Stepping Stone and on your ongoing journey to Slim Land.

However; on this journey things will happen and there is a high probability that you will fail with some things.

Failure can be viewed as the end or it can be viewed as an opportunity. I view failure as an opportunity.

Failure can be avoided, it can be reduced and you can learn from it; but you can never eliminate it.

When failure does happen, and for many of you it will, you have to understand that when it does happen it can provide you with a learning opportunity.

Make a mistake and Learn; or Give up?

Successful weight loss and successful long term weight management is about working towards an achievable goal; it is not about never failing.

Think how often all the people that you admire have failed?

Athletes, actors, politicians, artist, singers, writers, film directors, business people, our parents, friends and anyone who wants to achieve anything that is difficult.

Successful people don't give up just because things get difficult or because they fail at something. They may feel like giving up at times but they don't. I know because I have been there many times myself.

They keep their eyes on the long term objectives and the goals that they have; and they persevere until they achieve those goals and objectives.

And this is what we are going to do with your journey from Fat Land to Slim Land.

We are going to persevere with being successful and not let any obstacle, challenge, issue or person get in the way and prevent you moving on to the next Stepping Stone; and from there into Slim Land.

The thing about you being successful and overcoming adversity is that you need preparation and practice to do so.

The point about practice is that when you get to the real thing; the real thing is easier to do because of all the preparation and practice.

This part of the book is going to provide you with more of the information, advice and support that you will need to reach Slim Land and be able to stay there.

Note

The 2nd Stepping Stone is where the dieting organisations, fad diets, diet products and quick fixes all want to have a part of their business.

Real Estate on the 2nd Stepping Stone is at a premium

because so many people want to sell you their secret of successful weight loss, fast weight loss, easy weight loss, etc.

Depending upon the success of this book, I am sure that at some point someone will try to sell you the quick, easy and successful way to cross the 3 Stepping Stones.

Or, they will try to sell you the quickest route from Fat Land to Slim Land that will cut months off your journey.

What you need to understand is that if it was as easy as they make it out to be; then why do they have an 84% failure rate!

With the work that I do; I am trying to build something that actually does work and that has an above average success rate.

We can't achieve that with hype and big promises. We achieve it by being grounded in the reality of the situation and then working with it and changing it.

With all long term weight problems it takes time to fix them and to get to Slim Land. If you try to cut that time down, then all you do is that you reduce your chances of success. It is better to take a bit longer than you need; rather than trying to take less time than you need.

Regardless of how bad your weight problem is; it can be improved, resolved and better managed.

So let's get to it!

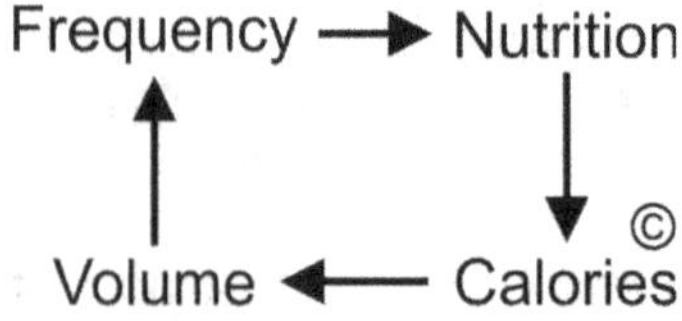

CHAPTER 12

The Diet & Weight Management Process

A diet and a weight management process are not the same thing.

A diet is about losing weight and often about quick weight loss.

Weight management is about maintaining weight within a range, and if necessary, losing weight or putting on weight to get into that range.

Diets usually have a short term focus, whereas weight management would usually have a long term focus.

Weight management becomes an integrated part of your lifestyle management. Whereas; it becomes very difficult to incorporate a diet, which has a focus on losing weight quickly, into your lifestyle management.

And when you look at what most dieters really need; they actually really need Weight Management and not a diet.

To live in Slim Land; you can't be reliant on diet products or prepared diet foods. Diet products and diet foods can and will have hidden ingredients that cause you to remain connected to Fat Land.

Diet products and prepared diet foods also carry a strong message that you can't really do this on your own; and they encourage you to remain in "the dieters' mentality".

It is the dieters' mentality that keeps you connected with Fat Land. In effect; its keeps a place open for you there for when you are ready to return from your visit to Slim Land.

To help you maintain the dieters' mentality; you will encounter lots of subtle media pressure to compare yourself with models that only exist as computer enhanced creations of feminine beauty.

You will see celebrities who will encourage you to use a certain diet or diet products. You will encounter teenagers with young skin who will encourage you to use certain beauty products to remain youthful and desirable.

You will see older celebrities and actors with studio lighting that hides every age line; encouraging you to buy and use certain products to keep yourself looking desirable and beautiful. *If you actually see these people in real life you will see that they age just like you and me.*

They are using your fears, your anxieties, your lack of confidence and self-esteem; and your desire to look and feel better; to seduce you to give up your control and to rely upon them for a better quality of life. And they cannot actually really give it to you.

I am not saying that you should not use beauty products and look after your body. What I am saying is don't be seduced by things which will take you off track and get you going in the wrong directions.

The same is true for diet clubs, gyms and exercise classes. Use them for your achievable goals but ask yourself whether the prize you seek is within their gift or yours?

Remember what I said about tranquilisers: Use a diet and diet club like someone would use tranquilisers; they can help you get out of a depression but they cannot keep you out of one permanently. Sooner or later you have to take over and do it under your own steam.

If you are over reliant on them; you won't be able to go it alone.

Think of this:

> Do you find diet clubs in Fat Land or in Slim Land?
>
> They go where the customers are and they are all in Fat Land.

The diet industry has spent a great deal of money trying to make us believe that there are simple and easy ways to lose weight.

It is likely that over the years you have been conditioned to think that all these problems can be fixed in easy and simple ways.

Once they have you convinced of this, then they sell these ways to us; regardless of whether they work or not.

What I am going to do with this section of the book is to give you certain fundamentals which I think will help you with the dieting process and also with the weight management process.

I am hoping at this stage, you realise that on the 2nd Stepping Stone, you are going to be focused on Weight Management as I described it early in this chapter and not on losing weight quickly by dieting.

There are just 4 fundamentals that you need to understand and practice with food and dieting; as these are the cornerstones of getting to Slim Land and living in

Slim Land.

1. Nutrition.
2. Calories.
3. Volume
4. Frequency - Food Flow Rate

If you can understand and work with this simple process then you can become successful with Weight Management.

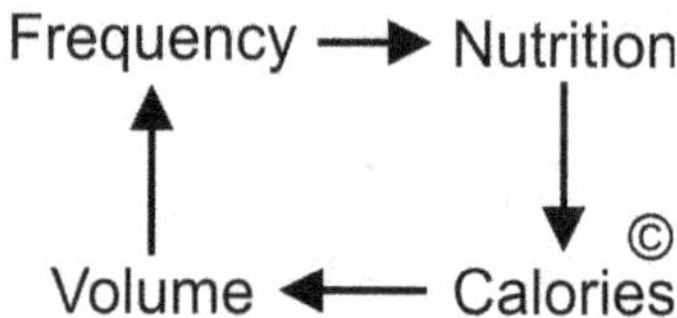

Now you don't need to become an expert on nutrition or calorie counting. What you need to understand is the relationship and balance that exists between these four components of food and healthy nutritious eating.

Understand how to use that balance and you will become a successful person who moves from Fat Land to Slim Land and stays there.

We will be using The Dieters Scale and Zones to help you understand weight management in a user friendly way, which you can use regardless of any diet that you follow.

> These simple principles can be applied to any diet and any diet product.

At this stage you should have a clear idea, or be getting a clearer idea, of what diet plan, programme or self-diet that you are going to use or follow.

And you should begin to understand what the diet is promising you and what it can really deliver.

Remember that there is an 84% failure rate with dieting for a reason.

> Marketing promises are easy to make. Achieving a higher than average result with people who use a diet or weight control plan is much harder to achieve and maintain.
>
> This is what we are after with The Human Algorithm® Approach; higher success rates which become higher long term success rates.

One of the things that you have to watch out for is the healthy diets and healthy foods which are not actually as healthy as you are being lead to believe.

There are lots of false, misleading and downright outrageous claims made for foods, drinks, supplements, dieting aids, over the counter medication, exercise equipment and items that contain things such as magnets, crystals and other totems.

Before we look at Nutrition, Calories and Volume I want you to understand and keep the following information with you.

CHAPTER 13

Frequency = Food Flow Rate

Frequency is actually easy to understand. It is the frequency and consistency of the flow of food and drink that goes into your body. This means:

- How often you eat.
- How often you eat what you are eating.

The Food Flow Rate is actually something that your body needs to be consistent and it needs to be within certain boundaries. If it is not consistent and within certain boundaries, then it can throw a spanner into your dieting efforts and screw things up.

> Most dieters do the wrong thing with Frequency because the right thing seems to be counter intuitive.

People with weight problems do mess up their own bodies Food Flow Rate and this in turn messes up how their bodies manage, process and recycle the foods that they eat and drink.

If you are in the Amber and Red Zones on The Dieters Scale then the odds are that your bodies Food Flow Rate is out of balance and it will need to be restored or reset.

Doing this is quite straightforward and this is how you can do it.

These are my own must have's for a diet. I have found

that these simple things, consistently applied, do make a big different to dieters long term behaviours and their long term weight management success.

Dave's Diet must have's!

In my view you need to:

1. Eat regular meals.
2. Of regular types.
3. At regular times.

This process helps your body to trust that it will have food at regular times, of a certain quality and at consistent volumes.

If you lose that regular pattern then your body will adjust accordingly to the irregular pattern; and you will feel the effects of chaotic and inconsistent food consumption.

In my view you should always try to eat a good breakfast and not feel hungry within at least a few hours of eating. This helps to stop mid-morning snacking.

You should have a good lunch and also not feel hungry within at least a few hours of eating. if you have snacked and don't feel like eating lunch then what will happen is that you will snack in the afternoon and this will then have a knock on effect for your evening meal.

In the evening you should also have a good meal and not feel hungry within a few hours of eating. This helps to stop snacking during the evening and it helps you then avoid skipping breakfast the following morning; because you feel guilty about what you eat the previous evening.

Now you need to do this even if you don't really feel like it. This is because you need to establish a proper pattern of "eating consistently" which your mind and your body can trust will continue.

Eating the same amount each day but with an irregular pattern is different from eating it with a regular pattern. This can produce different outcomes although you are eating the same amount.

If you don't follow this simple process then you are introducing chaos into the process; and we know what chaos produces.

What you need to understand about this simple process is that if you eat a main meal; and breakfast, lunch and your evening meal are main meals; and you do feel hungry quickly, then there is something wrong with either the type of food or quantity of food that you are eating; or with both of these things; which you can then fix.

Personally I am not a fan of many of the breakfast cereals that have increased in number in recent years. I personally would not consider them to be a proper breakfast and the small volumes you need to consume to keep calories low are beyond many people. They also have far too much sugar and other crap in them.

The next thing that you need to do with food is this:

- Begin managing the food.

If you live on your own or in a household full of other people; you need to begin to manage your food. What this means is that you make simple and little changes by taking baby steps.

By the time that you actually begin the diet you have chosen, you should already have began the foundations of the diet by implementing it and practicing it. Once you are on the diet proper you can continue this as required.

What you need to understand is that you can stay on the preparation and practice stage for the diet proper, until you find that you can easily do all the other bits. Take as long as you need. Speed is not your friend at this stage so take it slowly.

If you have a family I would suggest that you try to avoid having to cook different meals for everyone as this just creates problems long term and it's stupid.

You want to avoid creating a new generation of dieters and most people can eat good wholesome foods.

Also because you are using a diet plan, your food doesn't have to be boring. Make it interesting and enjoyable to eat.

If your family is eating all the stuff that made you put on weight, then you have to ask if they should really continue with that. Unless of course you have got into the habit of eating all the food that they leave as well as your own. Mommy food disposals can take on a lot of extra calories!

What you should do before you go on the diet proper, is to experiment with Slim Land food. This will help you get used to the different taste and flavours.

The reason we would practicing doing this is that when

you do live in Fat Land, you have a Fat Land diet. And as a result of living in Fat Land you have developed a taste for Fat Land food.

You have to realise that many of the foods that help us to put on weight "taste great" and we become very used to the taste, flavour and texture of that type of food.

As you move out of Fat Land you don't have to lose great tasting food; but you do need to understand something.

You need to understand that you may have developed "the taste" for Fat Land foods because they often have extra fats, sugars and other additives that our bodies can get used to quite quickly.

As a result of this it will take time for you to lose the taste for Fat Land foods. These are the foods that have the extra hidden sugars, fats and other things that can get you into trouble long term; and make weight management very difficult rather than easy.

Don't let yourself fall into the trap of thinking that low sugar and low fat foods must be good for you. The reality is that we all need fats and sugars in our diets in order to be fit and to be healthy.

Your problem is that you are taking in too many calories that may be hidden or in plain sight; because of a chaotic and out of balanced weight management structure. This is what needs fixing and the food and the results will follow this.

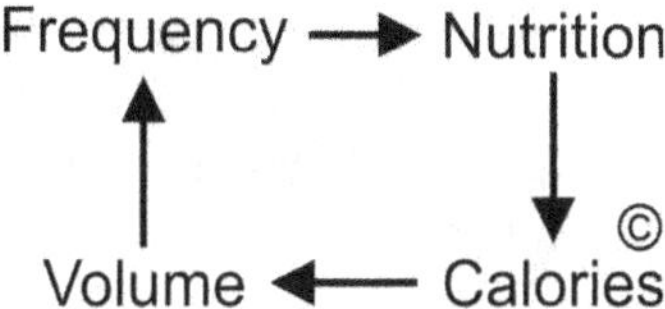

Now something else that you need to understand is that the same food does exist in both Fat Land and in Slim Land. Let's use pasta as an example.

Slim Land pasta will be the same base product and it will be cooked in the same way as Fat Land pasta. It is what is added to it as it is cooked and after it is cooked that alters things.

Fat Land pasta may have a very tasty highly flavoured sauce mixed in with it. It needs to be highly flavoured because Fat Land pasta eaters have got used to highly flavoured foods.

To achieve the high flavour, additives and other ingredients will have been added into the sauce. It won't be the pasta that is the problem; it's the sauce and the other things which get added to pasta.

Slim Land pasta will also have a sauce added to it that is very tasty. But a Fat Land person has got used to a sauce that is full of other ingredients and it does not have the same punch; so by comparison it can taste bland.

So you need to allow the time for your taste to change and be able to appreciate different and more subtle taste and flavours.

Here is a fundamental truth!

In Slim Land and in Fat Land people lie about foods.

In both places people will tell you that their food is healthy and good for you.

In both places they will tell you that their food is low fat, low sugar, low salt and so on. People and companies tell lies and practice deceptions in their marketing and in the promoting of the products that they sell and want you to buy and use.

Just because something says that it is low in fat does not mean that it is actually a "healthy food". Low fat can mean high sugar and other things that you don't want.

Low in sugar does not mean "healthy food" because if they are taking the sugar away they need to make it taste good by adding something else that you like; this may mean that it is high in fat and other things that you don't want.

Food marketing can be like a politicians promises. It sounds good and it can get your vote; but let's see what it really does over the long term.

> So don't be seduced by someone who is telling you that they sell food to people in Slim Land and you should buy it.

With all the different types of information that is around how on earth can you make sense of it all?

People will use different types of food labelling schemes, different types of healthy food labelling and different names to disguise additives that people want to avoid.

And then there is the guidance from the Government and the Medical professionals about what is and isn't good for you.

They can contradict themselves; one time they are saying that things like butter are harmful and that we should use margarine; then they say that butter is better for you than margarine???

Over the years I have heard all sorts of stupid things come out of the various organisations and Governments. And I have seen them do numerous 180 degree turns about things.

So I am going to give you my take on a simple system that you can use to help you with managing your diet and getting an appropriate balanced diet for your lifestyle needs. Please don't confuse this with any other system that you may come across as this is all my own work.

Dave's Guide To Food

To help you I am going to give you my guidelines. If you follow these guidelines they will help you avoid a lot of the crap.

What we need to get a handle on is the following:

1. Nutrition.
2. Calories.
3. Volume
4. Food Flow Rate = Frequency

In all foods Nutrition is important.

Nutrition is all the different components that your body needs to have in order to remain healthy and fight off infections and diseases.

All of us, without exception, need to eat fats, sugars, proteins and other nutrients, vitamins and minerals.

If we don't get enough Nutrition from our diets then we may need to supplement our dietary needs. This is where the different mineral and vitamin supplements that you see for sale come from.

Personally I do take a couple of supplements. I have done so for years and I will continue to do so. But I don't pay a lot of money for them and it doesn't matter if I miss taking them at times. I have chosen ones that work for me and give me an extra little bit of something that I think will help me.

What you need to understand about nutrition, is that it is possible, and it happens regularly, for someone to be very overweight and eat lots of food but suffer from a lack of Nutrition.

Calories and Nutrition are not the same thing.

We can use The Dieters Scale to help us understand more about Nutrition.

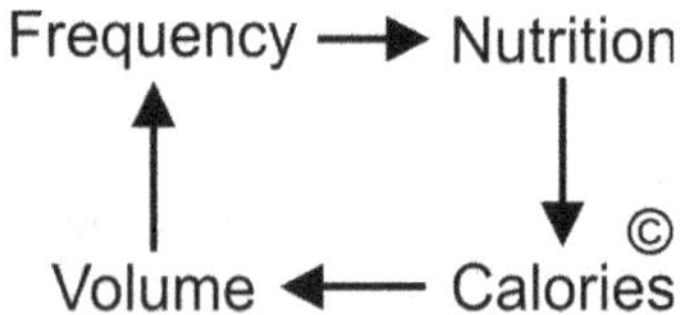

CHAPTER 14

Nutrition

Nutrition does not exist in all foods. Some foods have a good level of Nutrition and some foods have little or no Nutrition in them.

With all food and drink the level of Nutrition is a measure of the real nutritional items that are in it; like vitamins, minerals, fats, sugars, etc. These are things which our bodies need in order to work properly.

And all of these Nutritional levels will be in the ranges from; none to low (Red Zone); low to medium (Amber Zone) or medium to high (Green Zone).

With some foods our bodies can recycle the Nutrition from the food easily and from other foods it is more difficult.

Below we have A Dieters Scale showing Nutrition levels.

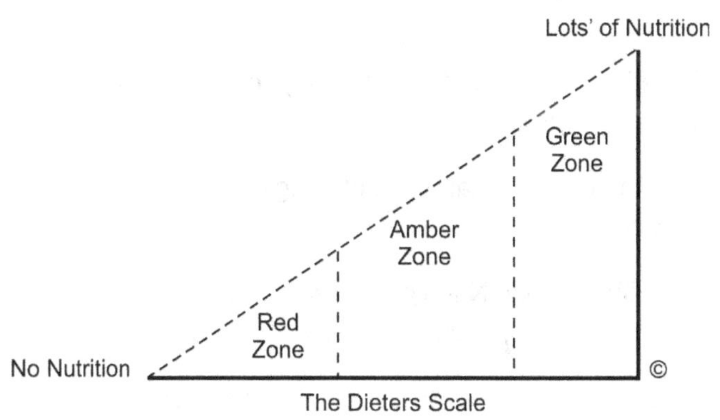

Green Zone Nutrition = Good nutrition levels.

Amber Zone Nutrition = Low to Medium nutrition levels.

Red Zone Nutrition = Little or no nutritional levels.

And this is how it works.

When we eat or drink foods we process that food in our digestive system. Our bodies then recycle the different minerals, vitamins and other things which it can recycle.

Our bodies are not 100% efficient and so we don't really know exactly how much of anything we do eat is actually recycled. Some of the Nutrition is recycled and some it can't be.

Also things like our overall health, the condition of our digestive system and other factors do play a part in this recycling process.

This is why it is important that we get your digestive system working better before you do go on any diet. It simply increases your chances of being successful.

So let's look at what types of things belong in the different Zones.

As examples of what types of things go into these Zones we would have:

Green Zone Nutrition = meats, fish, cereals, fruits, vegetables, yogurt, whole milk, cheese, eggs, etc.

When I am talking about meats, fish and cereals I am talking about unprocessed and uncooked foods. As these foods are processed and cooked the nutritional content and nutritional level can change.

Fast frozen/flash frozen fruit and vegetables tend to be OK but these will be unprocessed and not cooked.

> Amber Zone Nutrition = Bread and bread based products that are generally made quickly and in volume; yogurts that are processed.
>
> Processed foods that can keep on the shelves for a long time tend to lose their nutritional level with time.
>
> Fruits and vegetables out of season often have different levels from those in season.

As a general guide; food that is stored for a long period of time loses it nutritional level. Fruit and vegetables that are consumed immediately or soon after picking will have the highest levels.

> Red Zone Nutrition = Fizzy drinks, hot drinks, alcohol, processed cheese, fat free milk, processed sugar, many processed breakfast cereals, etc.

Now due to the way that the food industry works there are many, many different combinations of foods with varying degrees of nutrition. Some foods in one combination may fit into the Green Zone, others will fit into the Amber Zone and others will fit into the Red Zone.

Some food combinations, such as pizzas, may have a base which fits in one Zone and fillings which fit into another. So to make it easy you take an overall view of the thing that you eating.

Much of the food industry thrives on confusion and a lack of clarity. This is why getting a simple universal system that is easy to understand has not happened.

The point that you need to take away from this is that just because something can be eaten and someone is saying that it is healthy; this does not mean that it is Nutritious or that it actually has any Nutrition in it.

What you need to do it to make sure that your diet has sufficient Nutrition from the right Zones.

For example; you may have most of your Nutrition from the Amber Zone and make up the balance from the Green Zone. This would probably suit most people and produce a sustainable diet.

You may also consume things from the Red Zone but they will not contribute much if anything to your Nutritional needs. However; they will normally be high in Calories and so will quickly add Calories into your diet.

If you are eating most of your foods from the Red Zone and some from the Amber Zone then, over time, you can become Nutritionally deficient while eating lots of Calories.

Drinking lots of alcohol, for example, would be a Red Zone activity as it is Nutritionally deficient but high in Calories.

Becoming Nutritionally deficient may make you feel like eating more as your body will try to get the Nutritional things that it needs from what you are actually eating.

As you eat more; this in turn increases the Calories you take in and this in turn increases your weight; and it become a vicious cycle.

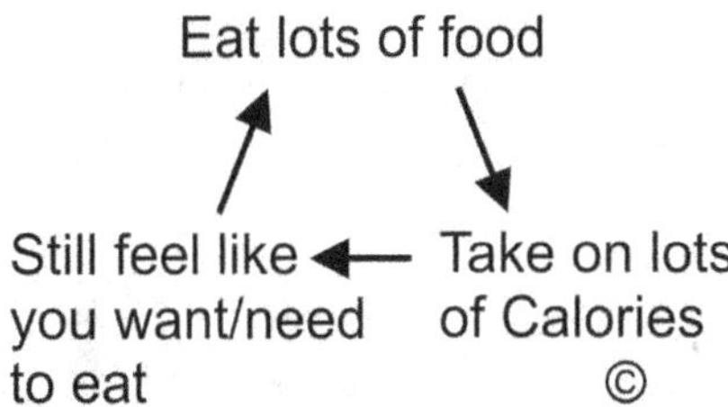

In simple terms: The more balanced that your eating is; the less Volume of food you will need to eat to give you the necessary Nutrition that you need to be healthy.

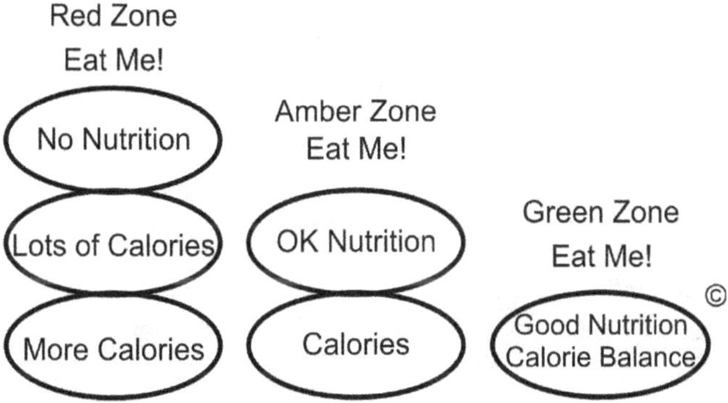

If you reduce the Volume of food that is required then this limits the amount of extra and unnecessary Calories that your body will have to process and recycle.

This in turn means that you put on less weight.

What you need to understand is this:

Green Zone foods have the best levels of Nutrition. You can only get certain types of Nutrition from Green Zone foods.

To satisfy your Nutritional needs you will need to consume more Amber Zone foods than Green Zone foods.

So if you don't eat enough Green Zone foods then the volume of food you need to eat from the Amber Zone needs to increase to try and compensate.

As the volume of food increases in the Amber Zone, Calories are likely to follow and you will consume more Calories as you try to get the Nutrition you need.

This is where the relationship between Nutrition, Calories and Volume comes into play.

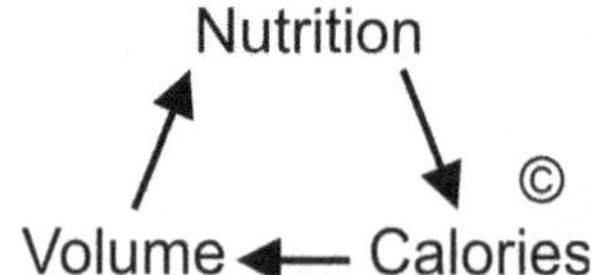

Consuming high volumes of Nutritionally deficient foods can still leave you deficient in the Nutrition that you need to be healthy.

These Nutritionally deficient foods can also leave you with thousands of Nutritionally deficient Calories.

And this is guaranteed to keep you in Fat Land.

So now let's look at Calories.

CHAPTER 15

Calories

Basically; Calories = Energy that is stored in foods.

Nutrition can be thought of like the engine and calories can be thought of like the fuel that goes into the engine.

We use Calories to give our bodies the energy that it needs to function, remain healthy and for us to do things with it.

Calories come out of the things which we consume in liquid and solid forms. For example; milk, cheese, bread, chips, pizza, cakes, burgers, etc.

Normally Calories come as part of a package.

For example; we grill some meat and eat it. The meat has Nutrition and it will have other components which we need to survive; it will also have Calories. That's the package!

As our bodies digest the meat, it is broken down into different components by our digestive system and our body uses what it can. What it can't use it will store and the waste product from the meat is pushed out of our bodies when we go to the toilet.

As we digest the Calories some will be used immediately by our bodies and some will be stored. This will be stored in our muscles and in our fat stores. We all have these.

Also what our bodies do is that they take different

amounts of time to digest different types and parts of foods. This means that the recycling process takes longer with things like nuts than it does with things like sweets.

So when we eat; a good strategy is that we consume a mixture of things that our bodies can recycle quickly and we also consume things which our bodies will recycle slowly.

The result of doing this is that our body gets the energy from what we have eaten; as it is digesting it over a longer period of digestion.

The amount of energy we need over the course of a day, a week, a month or a year; is dependent upon what activities we are doing, our climate, our lifestyles, our body type, our health; and how often we eat and what we eat.

What processes the food and drink we have eaten and drank is our digestive system. This is quite an efficient process most of the time but it can and does go wrong.

Our digestive system is full of different materials which work together to process, recycle and manage what we consume.

Our digestive system is like our own internal factory that takes in the food and drink that we consume and it recycles the various fats, sugars, proteins, minerals, vitamins and other things which we may need.

Just like any other factory; it requires that all the material it needs to work with are delivered in good order, in good time and in the right way.

Just like any muscle in the body; the digestive system can be fit and toned or it can be flabby and stodgy.

If we use the digestive system in the wrong way then it will try to adjust to cope with things. This ability to adjust means that sometimes things go out of balance and stay out of balance.

This is when we get digestion problems and other health problems.

The type, quality and volume of food and drink that we put into our digestive system will help to determine the health of our bodies.

This will also determine the amount of Calories that are stored as fat and how well our bodies will function with the various tasks that it has to perform.

> This means that what you eat and drink determines how well your body can function and how it is constructed and looks.

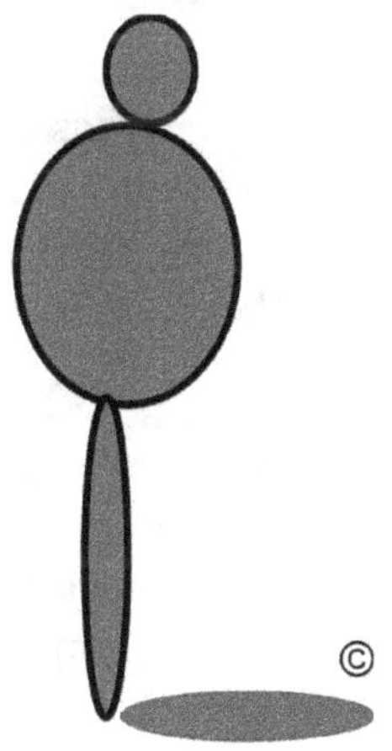

Chapter 16

The Dieters Scale for Calories

We will use The Dieters Scale to understand the Calorie impact different types of food have. It looks like this.

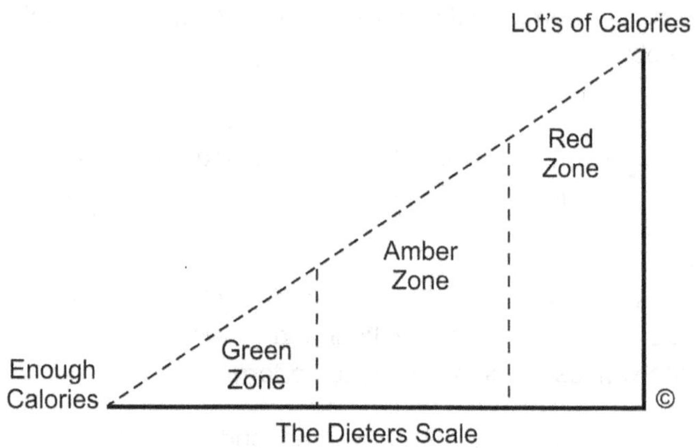

Green Zone Foods would be things like fruit and vegetable without any sauces on them. Natural yogurts (nothing added), milk, etc.

Amber Zone Foods would be things like bread, pizza's (generally better quality pizza bases and ingredients), certain pasta's, meats, cheeses and nuts. Burgers, fish & chips, fruit and vegetable with sauces, butters, creams, etc.

Personally I would include my homemade food. Things like fruit pies, bread rolls and cakes in the Amber Zone as I know exactly what is in them. Many yogurts and many fruit based drinks such as smoothies - I would put into this and the Red Zone.

Red Zone Foods would be things like store bought cakes, deserts (generally), sweets, candy bars, chocolates, many high calorie drinks, pizza's, burgers, fish & chips, fruit and vegetable with sauces, butters, creams, etc.

You will see that I have listed certain products in more than one Zone and this is because these can be made in different ways, with different ingredients, and this makes a difference as to whether they are in Amber or Red Zones.

The simple fact is that if you eat the same Volume of food from each Zone, then each Volume of food will have different amounts of Calories.

Once your weight is stable you can experiment with food from the different Zones. So no food is off limits to you and you are free to eat what you want.

However; there is always a simple reality that none of us can escape.

> If you want to eat too many Calories then this will eventually have an effect upon your body and how you look.

If you want to eat too much of the Red Zone foods then you may end up Nutritionally deficient and this can have long term health effects.

Most people's diets will balance out with a mixture of Amber and Green Zones with an occasional Red Zone.

If your Weight Management is chaotic then this will show in how you look and how you feel.

Chapter 17

An Alternate View of Calories

My own personal view is that we have become seduced by Calories and counting Calories. We portioned food into packets and we label that this food has (X) Calories.

We have been lead to believe that by consuming that food, that we now have those calories in our bodies and that our bodies have taken on those calories.

In reality Calorie counting is just a tool that should be used as a guide to help someone understand whether they are eating enough food. And in my view it has become misused.

> The reality is:
>
> It is your body's ability to recover the calories from that food and its ability to use those calories in your body that matters.
>
> And this will be an individual thing.

How calories are measured and displayed to us on a packet can be quite different from what your body can actually recover and use from it.

For example:

A bar of chocolate may have 500 calories. If you eat the chocolate we are lead to believe that we have consumed 500 calories.

We may have consumed something that contained 500 calories but that doesn't matter. What matters is how our personal factory (our digestion) will use those materials and how much of those 500 calories we can recycle.

> We don't recycle 100% of the calories in the chocolate bar.
>
> This is one reason why Calorie Counting can be erratic and produce different results from one person to another.

In reality that chocolate bar reaches our digestive system (our factory) and it has to be broken down into ingredients that our body can process. This recycling process uses some of that energy.

What also matters is how much time our body has to process and work on the chocolate bar.

If we have a lot of other things arriving in our factory then it will also be working on recycling those. If new things are coming into our factory then there is pressure to expel the chocolate bar and work on what else is coming through.

As a result of our "Food Flow Rate" our bodies can become more efficient at processing and recycling certain parts of the chocolate bar than others. And this is true for all sorts of foods and drinks.

What our body becomes efficient at processing may not be what we would like. Our choice has been removed once we put that food into our mouths and swallow it.

So if we are eating high volumes of the less desirable foods; then certain results are going to occur. We will continue to live in Fat Land and we will not be happy with ourselves.

If our Food Flow Rate is erratic, then it will affect the efficiency of our recycling factory (our digestive system).

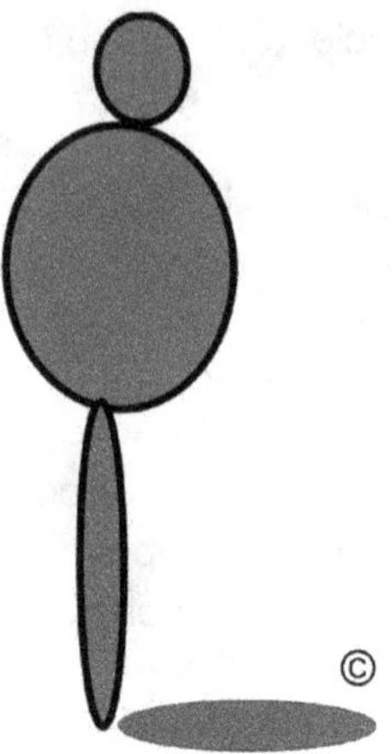

If we are eating more of the desirable foods and low volumes of the less desirable foods; then we can get a different result. We can live in Slim Land.

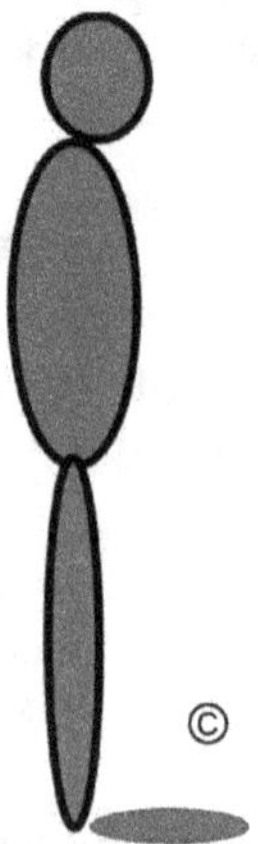

And this is what all dieting and long term weight control is about: Getting that right balance that we can maintain while living the life that we really want to live.

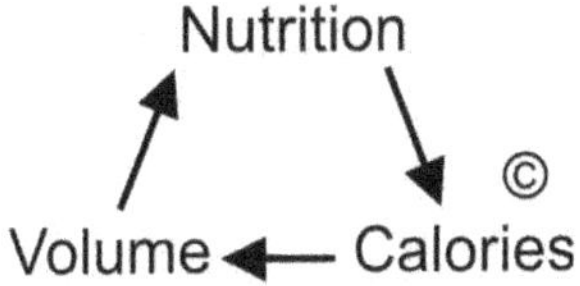

In my view Calories should only be a guide for foods and it should not be used by people with weight problems as "the way" of losing weight and managing their weight long term.

In my view it is the wrong tool and it brings with it the wrong expectations.

The tool we should be using is The Dieters Scale and applying this to the combination of:

Nutrition.
Calories.
Volume.
Frequency – Food flow rate.

It is this simple:

If your combination of Nutrition – Calories – Volume and Frequency; is in the Green Zone then you will find that <u>you don't</u> have a weight problem.

If your combination of Nutrition – Calories – Volume and Frequency; is in the Amber Zone then you will find that <u>you do</u> have a weight problem.

If your combination of Nutrition – Calories – Volume and Frequency; is in the Red Zone then you will find that <u>you do</u> have a weight problem.

So this tells you that you want to be more biased towards the Green Zone than you are towards the Red

Zone. This is illustrated on the following graphic.

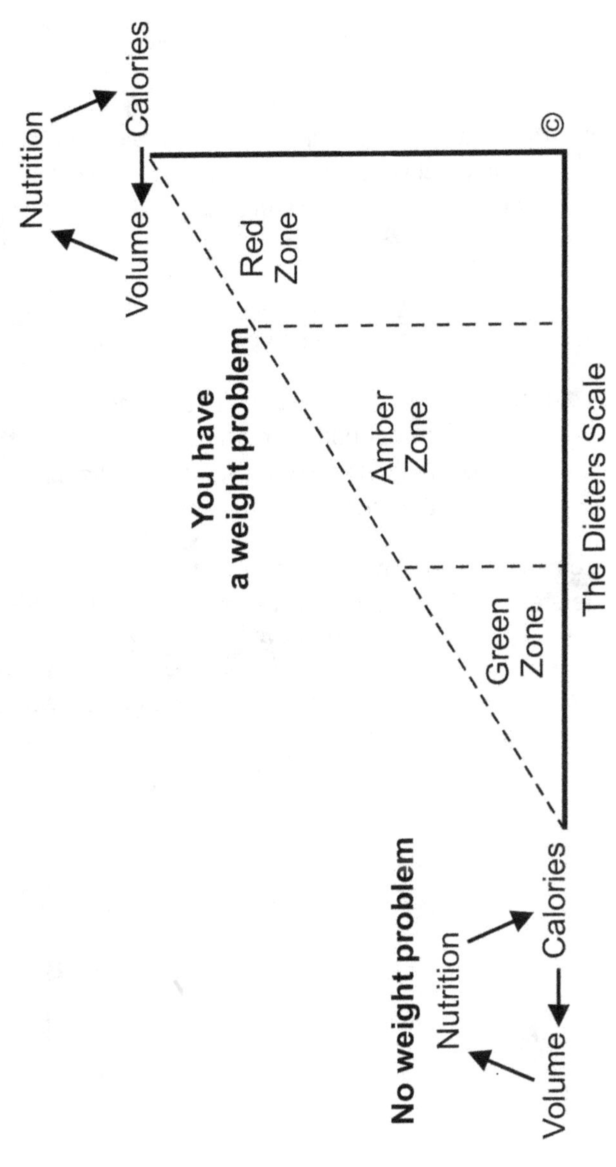
Nutrition
Volume
Calories
Red Zone
You have a weight problem
Amber Zone
Green Zone
The Dieters Scale
©
No weight problem
Nutrition
Volume
Calories

Chapter 18

Processed Foods

At this moment in time people have become exposed to food and drink that is new to our bodies. Because it is new, our bodies are either still adjusting to it or have not yet began adjusting to it.

We are encountering new combinations of foods, new structures of foods and new components of foods.

This causes problems, especially with processed foods as they can bypass our bodies' normal functions and cause us to consume more calories, faster and easier than we could in the past.

We can also take on new substances that we don't really understand and where we don't know what the long term effects of them are on the body.

To help you to understand processed foods better we will use The Dieters Scale.

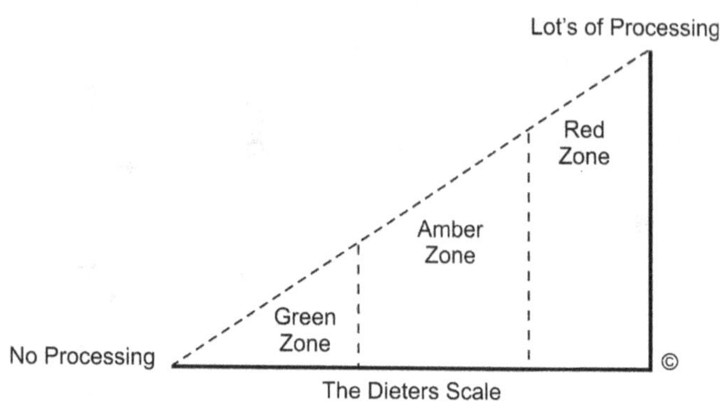

The Dieters Scale

Green Zone = Unprocessed foods.

Amber Zone = Lightly to medium processed foods.

Red Zone = Highly processed foods.

Green Zone would be things like a whole apple, a banana with the skin still on, an unpeeled orange, vegetables that are cooked from fresh and foods which are in their natural state.

Also fresh frozen vegetables, certain olive oils, honey, meat, fish, etc.

These are foods where very little or nothing at all is added to them. So there are no added salts, sugars, water, fats, flavour enhancers, emulsifiers, etc.

Personally I would add certain home cooked foods to this Zone as I personally know what is in those foods when I make them.

Amber Zone would be things like certain cakes that are made by your local baker and consumed on the day of baking. Things that need to be consumed on the day tend not to have preservers added but this is not always true.

Other things that would fall into the Amber Zone are certain takeout meals, cut meats like salami, certain ice creams, certain pizzas, certain burgers, etc.

Now this is my guide and some people would disagree with me about this but my point is:

There can be a big difference between the quality of products that are made at home, at restaurants, at shops, at factories and by food processors.

One restaurant may produce good food that fits nicely into the Amber and Green Zones. Another restaurant may produce the same things but use different ingredients and ways of cooking; and their food will fit into the Amber and Red Zones.

There is no easy to understand and use guide for this but you can use my various points to help yourself get better foods and to cut out foods that you didn't realise may be causing you problems.

If you eat only the cheapest and easiest foods, then you will find that a lot of what you eat will fall into the Red Zone. So what are Red Zone foods?

Red Zone foods would be things like certain burgers, certain sausages, certain pizza's, certain ice creams and things of this type, many sweets, chocolates, and items of this type.

Many of the cans and bottles of drinks, and the health replenishing drinks, do not have any natural or enough healthy ingredients in them; so I do question why we are drinking so many of them. Personally I would put most of them into the Red Zone.

Highly processed foods which are very cheap versions of more expensive and popular foods. Foods where you appear to get a high volume of food in a packet for not much money are often a guide to the quality of what is in the packet.

To be able to provide the more expensive foods at cheaper prices the main ingredients tend to be replaced by things like bulking agents. As a result you get less of the good stuff.

More and more foods are being sold on the basis of

"Tasting" like something or being "Flavoured" like something; rather than actually being what they are Flavoured to Taste like.

In my country I think that this is a problem!

So how do you balance this out?

To understand about balancing out your dietary requirements, with all the different foods that are out there, we will use Volume and we will cover this later.

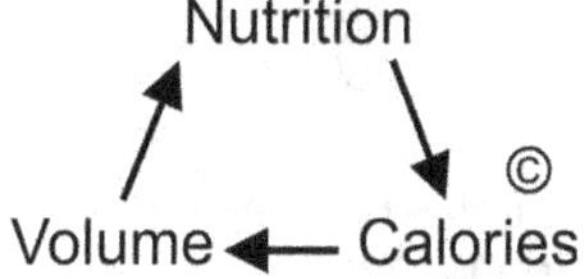

CHAPTER 19

Calories and Portion Control

Just about every person that I speak to about dieting and weight control replies with:

"It's all about Calories"

Let me challenge that point of view!

We have been lead to believe that women should consume about 2000 Calories a day and that men should consume about 2500 Calories a day.

This has become part of medical fact but it was never based on any serious medical studies.

My understanding is that this figure was thought up by someone as part of material that they were writing for a novel.

Over time this became part of Urban Legend and then medically acceptable. This was then built upon by the dieting industry and then became part of potion control and dieting products.

Now so many products have labels that tell you how many Calories you are going to consume by eating a specific amount of that product; and the assumption that people make is that these Calories will make up part of the 2000 Calories a day that they need.

In reality portion control and calorie counting is more suited towards making sure that someone gets a minimum daily amount of Nutritious food.

This is very important in countries where people have problems with the supply of foods and where people go hungry and die from starvation.

In the UK this was very important at times of war; such as during the second world war, when rationing limited the supply of food to the population. This restriction on the supply of foods continued until 1954 even though the war finished in 1945.

With potion control and calorie counting; the Government needed to understand the minimum amount of food that someone needed to have; in order to remain healthy. And be able to contribute towards the war effort in their different occupations. For example: Someone doing heavy manual labour V's someone working in an office.

It was a process that was controlled by ration books and coupons. You took these to the various shops and they exchanged coupons for rations.

In countries like Cuba this process is still used.

When someone is found not to be healthy consuming the allocated rations, these could be changed by doctors. Some people would develop things like Anaemia and they would be prescribed things like Guinness and red meats or extra rations.

So this process of Calorie Counting was about the Government getting the population to a minimum level of nutrition and calories; so as to maintain a satisfactory level of health. It was not about weight control for overweight people.

It has been adapted for weight control but I think that this is an ineffective way for most people to manage their health and weight.

When it is used by Governments you find that the population cannot easily supplement their diet by getting extra food. You simply can't get the extra food, so taking on extra calories is outside of your control.

In today's world the control has moved from Government to anyone with the money to buy food.

As a result of this shift, it is up to the individual now to make sure that they get sufficient food to maintain their good health. And to monitor the quality and Nutritional levels of their own foods.

> It's a case of: We are giving you the information and it's up to you make the right choices for you.
>
> You make the choice and you take the responsibility.

The problem is that we are not sufficiently educated in food management and weight management to do this.

We are still relying on external controls; where these external controls do not appear to be up to the job.

These external controls are the diet industry, the food industry, food regulators, Health Authorities and the Government. Also the Schooling system does not teach us things like Positive Lifestyle Management.

If they were doing the right job, in the right way; would we have the problems with weight that we now have?

In reality we have all been given choices; but they are

uneducated choices.

I want to help you get educated!

How it really works recap

Calories are an essential part of being able to live a healthy life. They are the fuel that we need to live a healthy life and to do things.

Calories come as part of a package with Nutrition and other items that may be attached to those Calories.

Some Calorie Packages are better than others. The Dieters Scale uses the Green, Amber and Red Zones to help you understand this.

As well as Calories we also need Nutrition to live a healthy life and do things.

To get the health balance right, we can't rely upon Calorie Counting because there are too many variables effecting our body's actual consumption and recycling of those Calories.

Over time our digestive system and our body's way of managing and processing the food and drink that we consume; can and does change.

Dieters often reach a point where their bodies digestive system and the way that they manage and process food and drink; becomes chaotic.

The result is that dieters have a chaotic and changeable dietary system and this impacts the way that it will manage and process the food and drink that they consume.

This is an individual process and no-one actually really knows exactly what is going on within any one else's body and how it is doing all of this.

How we find out how well someone's body is working and whether there is chaos; is we look at the result. For someone with a weight problem it's a case of how fat are they and how this is impacting their life.

When we are looking at someone's weight: If someone is in the Green Zone on The Dieters Scale then we know that there are fewer problems.

If someone is in the Amber and Red Zones then we know that there are bigger problems, more of them and that they are more difficult to deal with; and that they will take longer to deal with.

So let's see how Volume fits into this and how you can use this to help you with Calorie Counting or to replace Calorie Counting and portion control.

Volume is about how much fuel you really need to put into your body engine to run the engine. And to do the things you need to do; regardless of the actual Calories that you may count on a packet.

When you put fuel into a real engine this is the only place that fuel can be taken from.

Your body is different from this because your body's engine can take fuel from other places, other than the fuel tank.

Your body will take fuel from what is being processed in

your digestive system, it will take fuel from your muscles, and it will take fuel from your different fat stores. It will do the same with Nutrition.

Your body will use whatever fuel and Nutrition is the easiest and most efficient for it. You can't control this.

What you can do is to influence it and you do this by your Lifestyle Management and Weight Management.

You can really only influence things over time and you can change things over time. This "over time" approach produces sustainable results that can accurately and honestly be measured.

If you try to influence things too quickly, all you do is you introduce chaos or you increase the chaos that already exist.

When you try to do things quickly it can look as if you are achieving results in the short term but you won't be able to sustain them; and we don't want this!

So you can see how the pieces of the dieting puzzle come together and work. With this knowledge we can change the results that you have been getting and get better results that can be sustained long term.

So how can you use Volume to help you be successful with Managing Calorie?

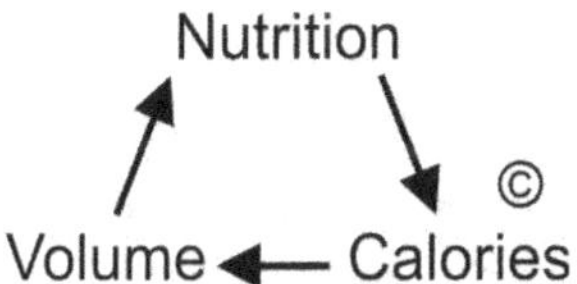

CHAPTER 20

Using Volume to Manage Calories

In the graphic below there are 3 cups. Anyone can see and understand that these cups are the same shape but of different sizes.

This means that if we were to fill each cup to the exact top with rice; that each cup would contain a different Volume of rice.

If we were to then cook and eat the rice from each cup in turn, we would feel either hungry or full after eating the contents of each cup.

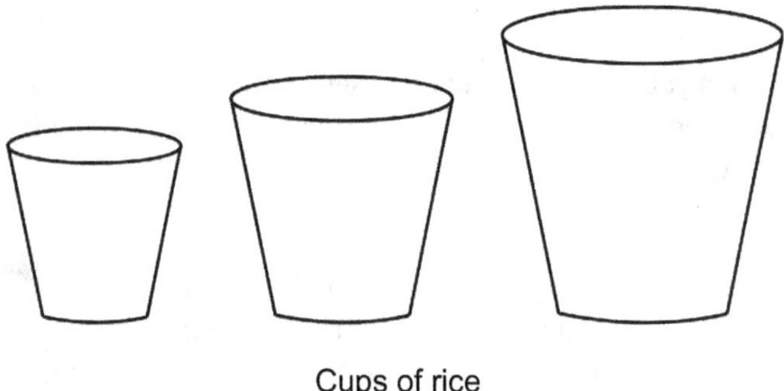

Cups of rice

If we eat from the smallest cup each day and we lost weight over time; then this would indicate that we are not eating enough. The overall Volume of food is not enough to sustain our weight.

If we eat from the second cup each day and we lost weight over time; then this would indicate that we are not eating enough. The overall Volume of food is still not enough.

If we eat from the largest cup each day and we lost weight over time; then this would indicate that we are still not eating enough. The overall Volume is not enough.

So it is not about the size of the individual cup itself; it is about how much Volume of rice that we need to maintain <u>our</u> weight and <u>our</u> health.

Now if we added something else into our diet. Let's say fish.

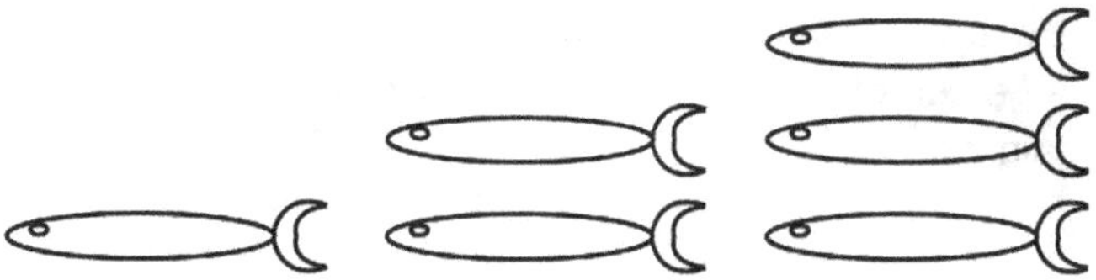

If we know that we lose weight regardless of what size cup of cooked rice we eat, then we may as well eat the largest one as we don't want to lose weight.

Now we can begin to add fish to our rice.

We begin by eating 1 fish and our rice but we continue to lose weight. The overall Volume of food is still not enough.

Then we begin to eat 2 fish and our rice and we do not lose any more weight. We now know that we are consuming enough Volume of the rice and fish to stop losing weight. The Volume is correct!

Just to be sure, we decide to check and so we begin to eat 3 fish and the rice. Nothing happens for weeks.

As we continue to eat the 3 fish and rice we begin to notice that our clothes are a bit tighter. We are putting on weight because we are consuming too much Volume.

We now know that the overall Volume is now too high and we are now putting on weight.

As we don't want to put on weight, we reduce the Volume of our food to 2 fish a day with the large rice.

Initially we may feel a little hungry because our body has got used to having too much food. But over a couple of weeks this feeling goes away and we gradually lose the extra weight.

We now know that when we maintain our diet at the large cup of rice and the 2 fish we do not lose weight or gain weight.

The Volume of food is correct!

So for this particular food mix and the activities we are doing; this is the correct volume that we need.

Now let's say that we wanted to eat more fish and vary it. How would we adjust this?

Well we know that 3 fish and the large cup of rice makes us put on weight because it is too much Volume of food.

So we eat the 3 fish and we change to the middle cup of rice, which has less Volume of rice. Our weight stays the same over a period of time.

The Volume of food is correct!

To check that this is correct we decide to keep eating the 3 fish but change to the small cup of rice. Over the course of the following weeks our weight goes down.

And from this little experiment, we know that the Volume of 3 fish and 1 small cup of rice are too little.

The Volume of food is too small.

So this means that we now have a choice with the Volume and Selection of foods. And this allows us to have more rice one time and more fish another time.

We can have the middle cup of rice and 3 fish; or we can have the large cup of rice and 2 fish.

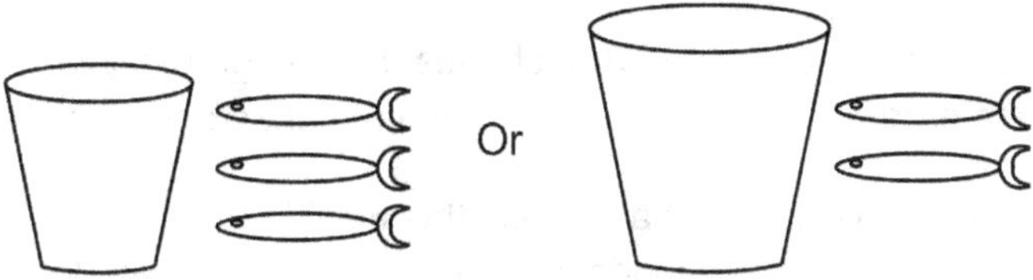

Either of these combinations gives us the right Volume of this food. Our weight stays stable and it neither goes up or down.

And this is the simple principle of Volume. We don't have to count Calories; we simply adjust the Volumes of the different foods that we are actually eating; until we get the right balance.

If we can't get the right balance with the volumes of food then we shift to another Zone.

For example if you are eating Red Zone high Calorie foods and you can't get the Volume right; then shift to lower Calorie foods in the Amber Zone and you should be able to get it right.

What you need to understand is this simple truth:

All successful dieting and weight management is about trial and error until you find what works for you. Then once you have found it: Apply it consistently.

Chapter 21

Burgers, Fries & Pizza

What happens if we were to change the food items to a more current dieting style for many of the people with weight problems?

Let's say that we had French fries, hamburgers, pizza, ice cream, fizzy drinks, fresh fruit, tea/coffee and water.

Now if this was all that we eat, this would not be a healthy mixture of foods. But let's see what we can do with this. So let's follow our simple process.

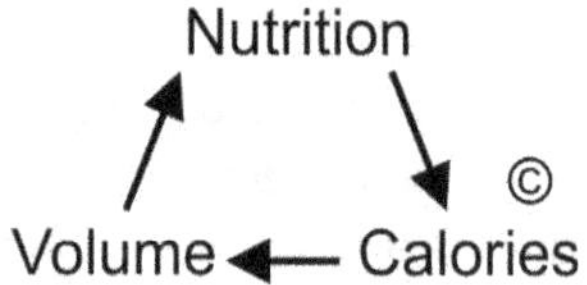

This food would mostly be in the Amber and Red Zones for Nutrition.

This food would largely be in the Amber and Red Zones for Calories.

The exception would be the fresh fruit which would be in the Green Zone for Nutrition and for Calories.

Now anyone who has a weight problem and who has a diet like this is going to be in the Amber and Red Zones on The Dieters Scale.

So let's see how the NCV Guide helps us to work with

this diet to manage the Calories and improve Nutrition.

Let's start with the Nutrition.

The food is: French fries, hamburgers, pizza, ice cream, fizzy drinks, tea/coffee, and water. These would go into the Amber/Red Zones for Nutrition. This is because the Nutrition will vary and much of this food could have little or none.

The fresh fruit would go into the Green Zone as different fresh fruits have different Nutrients in them and these are highest in the fresh fruits.

So the graphic below shows our relative Volumes of Nutrition that we are eating.

Nutrition Volume

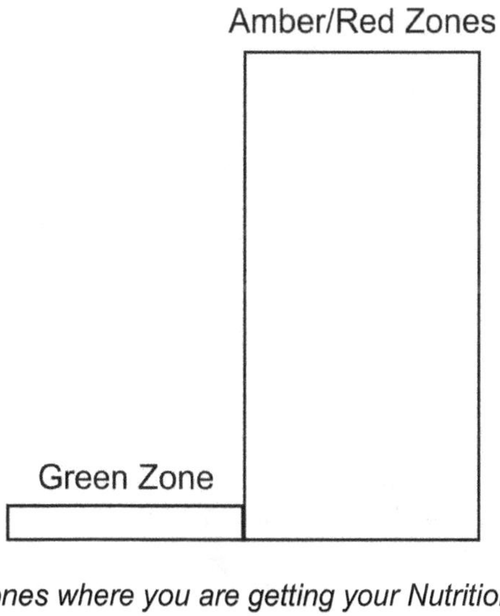

The Zones where you are getting your Nutrition from.

Let's say that this is your normal diet that you have had

for a long time and that you are overweight.

A diet like this over a long time will reduce your bodies Nutrition; unless you eat a lot of it. So to get the right level of Nutrition, in the way that you are doing it, requires a higher Volume which will cause you to take on more Calories.

Let's see where the Calories are in this food.

Calories Volume

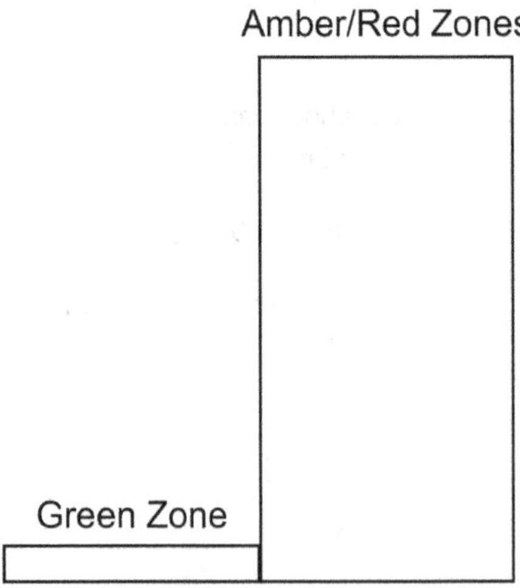

Amber/Red Zones

Green Zone

Virtually all of the Calories are in the Amber/Red Zones.

The Calories are mostly in the Amber and Red Zones.

And we know that the food is high in Calories in the Amber Zone and higher still in the Red Zone.

And if we looked at where the "Volume of food to give us the desired weight" was, we would find that the Volume of food that is being eaten is in the Amber and Red Zones, so we are eating too much Volume of these foods.

Volume of Food Eaten

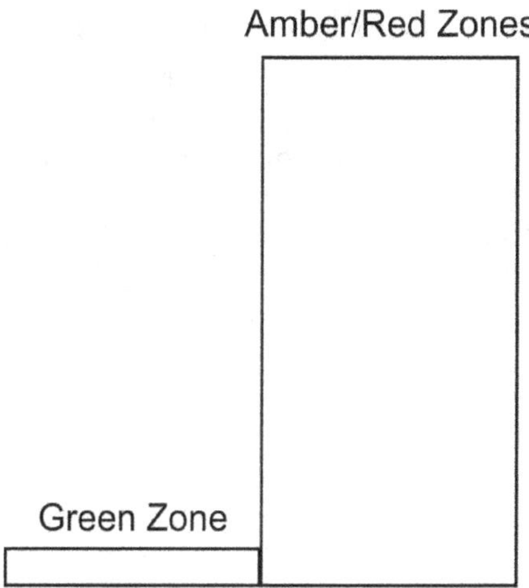

Most of the Volume being consumed is in the Amber/Red Zones.

And on The Dieters Scale; where would you be?

In the Amber or Red Zone!

So you can see that The Dieters Scale helps us to begin to understand the structure of a weight problem.

It also helps us to begin to understand our own weight problem in another way.

Once we have this understanding and knowledge we can then begin to do something different.

We can begin to see how we can influence that structure to achieve the results we want!

So how can you use Volume to help you “Manage Your Calories”, even with a diet like this?

Well hopefully you would be following The Stepping Stones Approach. And you would be in the Preparation phase, and you would be looking at practicing with your diet before you actually begin the diet proper.

If you just try this as a short cut it won’t work for you long term but let’s see what we could do if you were following the Fat Land to Slim Land plan.

CHAPTER 22

Adjusting Your Diet & Managing Calories

To refresh your memory the diet we are working with is: French fries, hamburgers, pizza, ice cream, fizzy drinks, fresh fruit, tea/coffee and water.

And we know that this diet is out of balance; and the person who has this diet is overweight and in the Amber or Red Zone on The Dieters Scale.

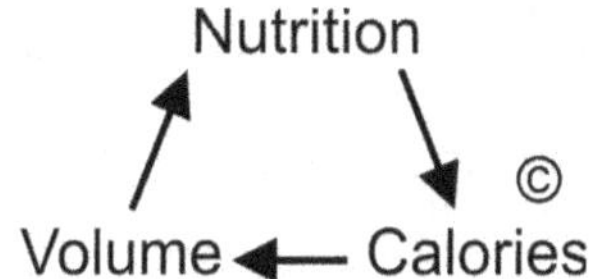

For the purpose of this exercise we will assume that you are overweight; that your weight is stable but it can vary a little.

We know that the Nutrition in what you are eating; and that the Nutrition that your body needs to maintain itself; is probably out of balance.

In any event if you were to increase the Volume of Green Zone Nutrition this would be a good start and it would help you move in the right direction. So let's do that!

1. Increase the Volume of Green Zone Nutrition and maintain this increase. You can do it a bit at a time but keep to the new Volumes.

   So this would be an increase in the fresh fruit and perhaps introducing fresh vegetables. Avoid switching to things like smoothies as a replacement.

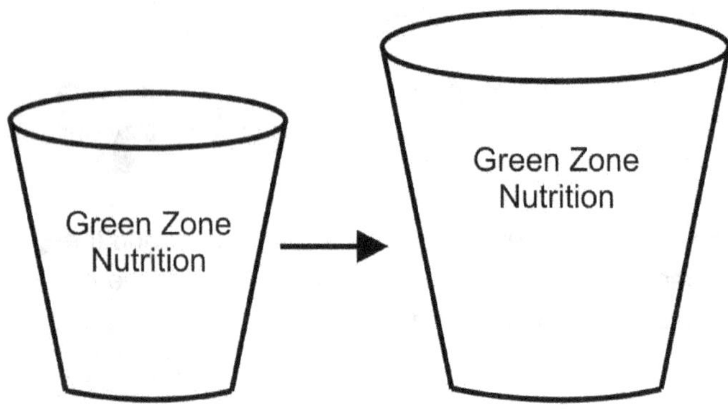

1. Increase the Volume of Green Zone Nutrition.

The next thing to do, would be something that you could probably do easily without really noticing it at all or very much.

2. Decrease the Red Zone food and drink you are eating and drinking and move this Volume to the Amber Zone.

Just by making slight decreases, regularly over a period of weeks, it will make a difference.

Things like fizzy drinks are an easy thing to reduce as many people just get in the habit of drinking them. They provide you with fluids but they often have lots of sugar in them and other things are often added that you really don't want. I personally would include Sports drinks in this.

Switch more to the tea/coffee or water. Watch out that

you don't add lots of sweeteners or cream to your hot drinks.

Changing pizza toppings, reducing the amount of olive oil and other oils (pizza's don't really need oils; I know because I make my own). Changing to a higher quality proper dairy ice cream, removing things like mayonnaise from burgers and changing sauces can all make a difference. Many of these are hidden Red Zone foods that you won't really miss.

Shifting the Volume from one Zone to another Zone has the effect of Reducing the Calories that you are consuming but maintaining the Volume.

By increasing the Nutrition and maintaining the Volume it is less likely that you would notice any real difference.

The Red Zone food will have little or no Nutrition but lots of Calories, so switching to the Amber Zone food increases your Nutrition while reducing your extra Calories.

This process makes it easier for you!

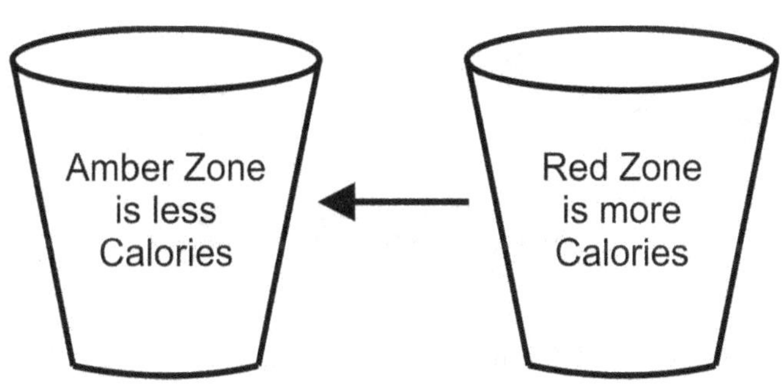

This simple process lets you adjust things slowly.

Doing these 2 simple things would begin to make a difference. It would be slow but this is what we want as your body has not had a chance to settle yet.

Now imagine if we repeated this process again once you got used to the first change?

Then we repeated it again, and again until you got to the point where everything related to your diet and how your body worked was more balanced.

You would get to where you wanted to get too without all the stress and drama that your conventional diet has and you would achieve more.

This simple process is sustainable, whereas the normal way that people approach dieting, with large sudden changes, is much less sustainable.

If people adopt this approach we can increase the number of people who successfully manage their weight problem and improve their lives.

The number of people who live in Fat Land will reduce and the number of people who live in Slim Land will increase.

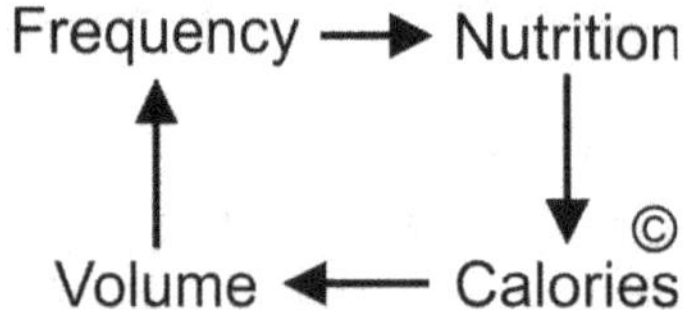

Once you have the right knowledge, achieving this

becomes a simple process!

Gradually you would make the changes to your Lifestyle Management. This would be things like your stress management, making time for yourself and the other things which we looked at for the 1st Stepping Stone; which was Preparation & Practice!

If you were to Prepare & Practice this stuff before you began your diet proper; how much easier would the diet proper be once you began doing it?

CHAPTER 23

Getting The Body Stable And Prepared To Go On The Diet Proper

If you follow the advice that I am giving you in this book, you will get to the point where your body becomes stable.

While you are waiting for this to happen, you will be able to begin adjusting the other aspects of your life that also need to be improved, to help your dieting experience be better.

My experience is that it takes about 3 months for someone's body to become stable and maybe longer for some other people who are more chaotic.

Getting your body stable is a part of the process that you can't actually rush. If you try to rush it then you will find that you just fall off the Stepping Stones and end up back in Fat Land.

If you get impatient and you try to push things to go faster; all you do is that you introduce chaos into a process that requires stability. When you do this all that happens is that you have to start the 3 month clock again.

If you get impatient and you go on the diet proper and you think that you have it cracked because you lose weight; well think again as you may be able to trick you mind but you cannot trick your body. Avoid the disappointment and wait until the right time.

If it was me doing this, then I would put a note in my

diary of when I began the 3 month stability stage and then review how I was feeling and whether I was ready to diet proper at that time.

If I wasn't I would diary more time and just continue to practice the necessary diet things to get and keep my body stable. And I would continue to practice the other lifestyle management things; like stress control that we talked about earlier in the book.

This in itself will usually begin to produce positive results for many people.

You have to constantly remind yourself of what it is that we are going to achieve here:

> What we are going to do here is to get you out of Fat Land and help you across the Stepping Stones and into Slim Land. Once you are in Slim Land we want you to be able to continue to live there.

To achieve this, enough things need to alter within your life and with your weight management processes for you to be able to get to Slim Land in the first place.

While you are waiting for your body to become stable there will be plenty of other things for you to prepare and practice.

Take this time to begin to practice and even change the way that you are actually doing and managing things.

This is the best time to do this because you haven't gone on the diet proper yet and so you haven't got all that stress.

CHAPTER 24

Achieving Stability And Moving On To The 3rd Stepping Stone

Let's move forward in time and say that you are now 3 months or more into your preparations and practices for the diet proper.

Well done!

If you have done the things that I suggested then you will have prepared yourself in a great way to be successful with this.

If you have been doing what I suggested and you are following and using the information; then you should be feeling better than you did at the beginning.

Now remember all the different things which I have told you; and keep reading through this book and taking note of the different information and advice.

As you move on to the diet proper it is important that you don't put yourself under pressure to achieve fast and consistent results.

If you do put yourself under pressure to achieve fast and consistent results, then all you are going to do is to reserve your place in Fat Land and make sure that you get back there quite fast.

Just take it one day at a time and do the things that you need to do on this journey.

If you have prepared in the right way, you will have practiced what to do when you have a bad day. So when a bad day happens, and it will happen at some point, then you will know what to do and how to handle it – Follow your plan when things go wrong as this will help you.

Whatever happens once you are on the diet proper, it is important that when something does go wrong (and it will) that you take a step back and manage it.

You might feel the compulsion to revert to what you would normally have done in the past; but take a step back and manage it.

If you can't take a step back and manage it and things go horribly wrong; don't worry - Learn!

Look at what happened and how it happened. What would you have changed to achieve a different result? Then remember that the next time.

Remember that you did not get into Fat Land and take up residence in Fat Land by just making one or two little mistakes over a weekend.

Getting into Fat Land was a process that you worked on, diligently, over a long period of time.

That process had a lot of little steps that took you there over a long period of time.

The following diagram illustrates this.

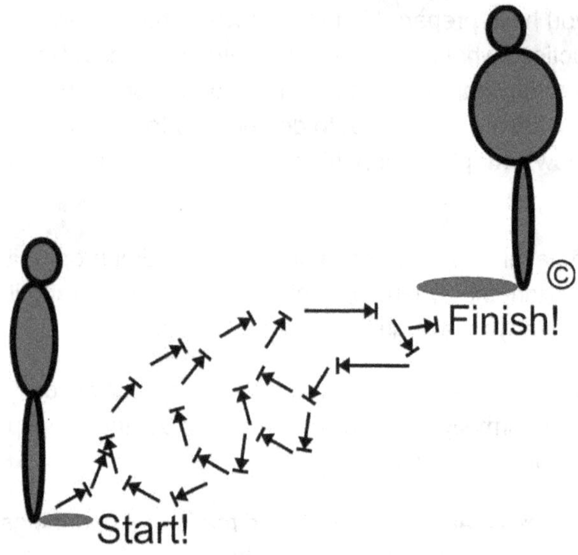

And what we want to do is to reverse that process and take a lot of little steps, over time, to get you out of Fat Land and into Slim Land.

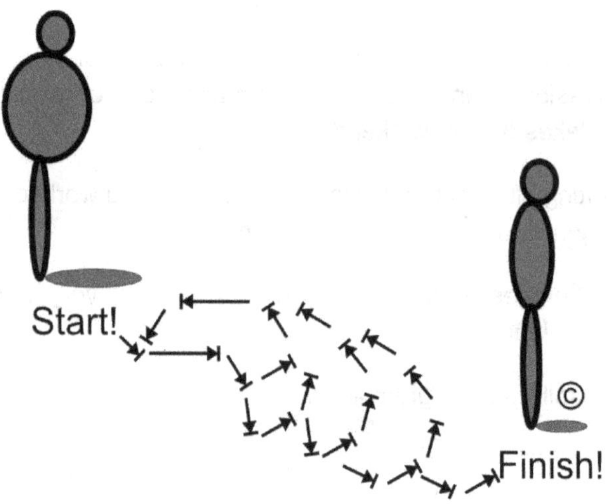

A major mistake that most dieters make is that they have been educated to think of weight loss as a straight line process.

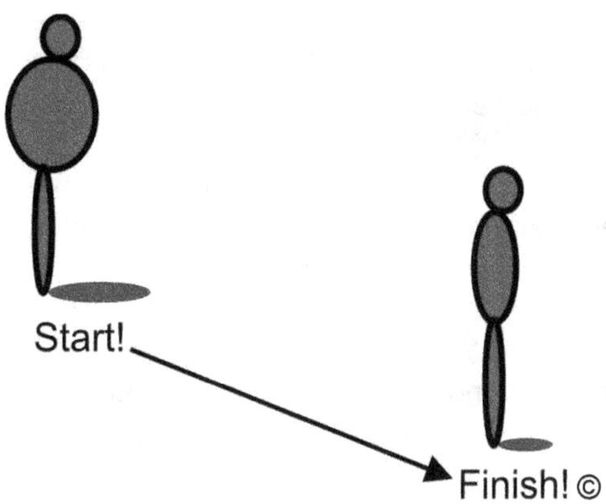

It's a false belief system that says that you control everything and that if you do the right things you can lose (X) lb's a week until you reach your target weight.

As I say in my book: The Perfect Life Diet For Imperfect People With Weight Problems; your body never got the memo!

You can influence how your body works over time and you can influence this in positive ways; if you do the right things, in the right way, at the right time, for the right reasons.

If you work with your natural processes, then you can coax them to begin to do what you want them to do.

If you do it the right way then your body will begin to produce the positive results that you want. And you will be able to maintain those results.

CHAPTER 25

Weighing Yourself – How Often?

Before we move on to the 3rd Stepping Stone I want to give you another little warning about weighing yourself.

So many people twist themselves into knots weighing themselves daily or weekly and for most of them this is unnecessary and counter-productive.

My view is that you should not weight yourself daily. Perhaps do it once a month and use other methods to give yourself a guide to how things are going.

Let me explain.

Your weight will vary throughout the day, week and month. Eating, drinking, moving around, the weather, going to the toilet and your choice of clothing all affect your weight and your body mass.

As you get hot or cold and as you move around, your body moves fluid into and out of your muscles and towards and away from your skin.

Your body and how it behaves and responds to different situations is all Dynamic. This means that it may be stable in one set of circumstances and conditions but that it can change and alter as these change.

Because of this Dynamic behaviour you can only measure things like your weight, body mass, physical dimensions, body fat, and any other way; by doing so over time and seeing what the Trend in measurements are over time.

That is:

Over time, is the trend that your weight's going up; is it holding steady; is it going down?

> Over time, are you feeling better than you did when you began this?
>
> Over time, are you looking better than you did when you began this?
>
> Over time, are you managing your Lifestyle better than you did when you began this?
>
> Over time, are you managing your food better than you did when you began this?
>
> Over time, is your weight management better than it was when you began this?
>
> Over time, is your weight more stable that it was when you began this?
>
> Over time, are you feeling happier, more in control and more positive about your future?

These are the types of ways that you should really be judging how you are progressing and what you are achieving.

That little indicator on the weighing scales is not the way that I would choose and it may be your short cut back to Fat Land. *I would suggest that you go back to point 29 in the 1st Stepping Stone section and read that again.*

Now we are going to move on to the 3rd Stepping Stone: Positive Lifestyle Management.

The 3rd Stepping Stone

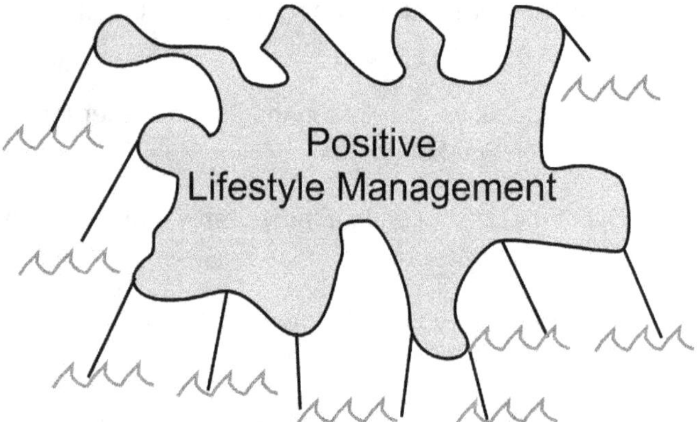

CHAPTER 26

The Common Purpose

What is a Common Purpose?

A Common Purpose is that your actions, motives and desires all share something which is the same.

In this book I have been helping you to develop a Common Purpose that supports your moving from Fat Land to Slim Land and being able to live in Slim Land.

> Successful long term weight management and having the life that you want to have, is achieved by a series of things coming together with a common purpose.
>
> That common purpose is to get you from Fat Land to Slim Land. And for you to be able to take up residence in Slim Land and live where you want to live and how you want to live.

This is the Common Purpose for everything that I have been telling you in this book: From Fat to Slim in 3 Steps.

As you move from Fat Land to Slim Land a number of things will change. One of those things is that your Fat identity will begin to change to your Slim identity.

This is what happens on the 3rd Stepping Stone; you allow yourself to change from the person who lives in Fat Land to the person who is now going to live in Slim Land.

You will need time to get used to this new identity and so will the people that you know.

However; you are the one who needs to live with this new identity.

A new identity is not about being a completely different person. It is about changing the things about you that you did not like and changing them to the things that you do like or prefer more.

By doing things slowly and a little at a time, it means that the people who you come into contact with regularly don't tend to notice any sudden changes.

You will also find that those little consistent changes in the different areas of your life that you want to change; are easier to do and manage.

What we are going to do on the 3rd Stepping Stone is to simply do more of what you have already been doing.

So if you have got this far then you should be able to go all the way!

At this stage I would like you to remember my warning!

I have seen many people achieve success and I have warned them about the Unexpected things which can happen.

I have had to talk a number of people through the shocks and knock-backs that they experienced when someone close to them did something unexpected or something unexpected happened.

These things take you by surprise (even when you have prepared for them) and they can knock you off your feet, take away your control and leave you exposed and vulnerable.

These things can often happen just when you think that

everything is going great and when you have let your guard down with certain people.

These unexpected things can come from unexpected people and unexpected places.

Part of what is happening here is this:

You want things to change and you are doing something about it.

Other people have got used to things being as they are and they may actually prefer them like that.

Now you may have spoken to this person (or family) about what you are doing and they may have said great! And that they are all with you.

But your previous dieting history probably tells them something different.

Anyway the long and short of it is:

> That many people, including yourself, may want things to change; but they get used to them being as they are. So there are often one or more attempts to maintain things as they were or to take them back to how they were.

Now these attempts can seem illogical, mean, stupid, nasty and destructive; but they happen.

People have a variety of reasons for doing this and they include: They are scared, don't know how to deal with the new you, can't control the new you like they did before, don't want to lose you, etc.

The other thing that can happen is that you get scared.

You may not know how to deal with the new you, not feel

ready to deal with a problem that you know you need to; and all sorts of things.

It may even be that you thought that you would feel differently, think differently or somehow become a totally different person on your journey to Slim Land.

The reality is that we evolve from one way of being to another way of being and it takes time; we have to adjust.

Now I can't give you the answers to these problems, issues and challenges but I can help you to manage them.

And this is where all that Preparation & Practice that I was talking to you about for the 1st Stepping Stone comes into its own.

You should have put those things in place and practiced them.

It is these simple things from the 1st Stepping Stone that begin to create "The Common Purpose" that you need for the journey from Fat Land to Slim Land.

As you moved on to the 2nd Stepping Stone you should have continued to Prepare & Practice them and used them.

Doing this embeds that Common Purpose into your actions and your thoughts; and it influences how you begin to manage and control the things that happen to you; and around you.

And in the process of going on to the 3rd Stepping Stone and going on into Slim Land you will continue to use and develop that Common Purpose.

You will use the new skills that you have been developing; the new strategies that you have put in place; that you tried out and became familiar with, with all the practice I have been encouraging you to do.

When a problem, issue or challenge occurs; always take a step back and take another look at what is happening and why.

Avoid knee-jerk reactions.

If you need a little space and time then take it.

Don't let others push you into making the decisions or taking the actions that you will regret later.

Learn to say No!

In any situation you may not know the positive end result that you would want from that situation. That is OK; because you probably will know the negative result that you don't want. If you can't work towards something then work away from something.

I have helped people to deal with some very bad situations in their lives. I have always found that Preparation and dealing with things in manageable pieces without over reacting is the best way. Its' not always the easiest but it is the best.

You may not always be able to do this but the work that we are doing here will provide you with the foundations that you need to successfully do this in the future.

Hold on to your dreams and work towards making them a reality.

CHAPTER 27

Locking Things In Place

On the 3rd Stepping Stone you begin a process of locking things in place and leaving old habits and practices behind.

One of those things you will lock in place is your new weight management process and one of those things you will leave behind is dieting and going on a diet.

Remember that going on a diet and weight management are not one and the same. If you confuse these two things you will find it difficult and be wondering why things are not working out for you.

This is because a diet tends to be something that people do for a period of time and then stop; and revert back to their previous normal eating habits which have not changed.

Weight management is a process that you use to manage your weight to a level; and then you continue to use those same processes to maintain your weight at about that level.

Also as you use and develop the weight management process, you change your eating habits and practices and these become your new and sustainable eating habits and practices.

If you find that your weight and eating habits begin to drift, you can reassert your weight management process and re-establish your new eating habits and practices.

When this is done properly you find that you do not have to diet at all. What happens is that you notice that you have put on or lost weight and you want to adjust things back to the right weight level.

Because we are looking at weight in a different way; you avoid any sudden over reactions and you simply adjust your weight management process, so that over the coming weeks and months you move back to the right level.

This type of adjustment does not throw your body structures out of balance; it does not interfere with your digestive system or your bodies recycling processes.

We avoid the chaos and it becomes a simple, easy and constantly achievable process. And this is exactly what you want.

Positive Weight Management is a part of Positive Lifestyle Management.

It is about being Pro-Active and dealing with problems as you see them coming or as they occur.

Positive Weight Management is about taking responsibility for what goes into your mouth and the effects of that consumption upon your body.

Positive Weight Management is also about taking control of how you use food in different situations when you are feeling vulnerable, scared or unsure about what to do.

Remember:

> It's not about what you eat or drink. It's about what you put into your mouth in the first place!
>
> If it never goes into your mouth, you never give your power away to food and drink.

You can then influence how your body works, how it looks and how it behaves by what you put into it.

Once the food and drink is in your body, you can no longer control it.

This means that we can use our influence to achieve the long term control over how we look and how we feel.

Positive Lifestyle Management is how you move away from a life focused on your weight and the problems that this causes in your life.

Positive Lifestyle Management is about making some positive choices about your life; and then making those positive choices into a reality.

It can be challenging if you are not used to doing this but it is something that everyone is capable of doing.

To achieve successful results with your Positive Lifestyle Management we will use the same processes that we have been talking about and using throughout this book.

Once again we use The Dieters Scale to help us in this process as it is something that you are familiar with.

To achieve the life changes that you want we will use The Dieters Scale and apply the Green, Amber and Red Zones to the different issues, problems and challenges that life naturally brings to us.

As a starting point for you, you could consider the issues, problems and challenges that the questions in the first section of this book asked you. Those are potentially things that impact your weight problem, impact your life and impact how you feel about and view yourself.

Managing these different things is like managing a weight problem; there are right ways to go about it and wrong ways.

We want to get more things right than we get wrong.

The Common Purpose that you have been developing will also influence these things in a positive way. This is because it begins to develop Purpose and Direction in your life that you can use and which will influence you.

By applying The Dieters Scale we can see that other problems, just like dieting, have different degrees of complication and difficulty attached to them.

For example: If we were looking at Self-Esteem, Confidence and Motivation; we would recognise that some issues are small and easy to address and some are difficult and hard to address.

The simple ones belong in the Green Zone and the difficult ones belong in the Amber and Red Zones.

And when we want to address these thing and being to achieve positive results we don't want to apply a Green Zone solution to a Red Zone problem.

Because now we know that if the Zone of the problem and the Zone of the solution do not match; then this has a very high probability that it won't work; and that we are just setting ourselves up to experience failure.

To break all these different problems down into manageable bits, we will combine the help that The Dieters Scale can give us, with The Stepping Stones approach.

If a problem is in the Red Zone we are unlikely to be able to jump from the Red Zone into the Green Zone.

So we begin a process of moving out of the Red Zone and into the Amber Zone.

Then we move out of the Amber Zone into the Green Zone.

Then we move to where we want to be in the Green Zone.

So we take a series of baby steps which have a Common Purpose: To take us in the direction of the positive result we want to achieve.

If we make an error and we put the problem in the wrong Zone, then we go up a Zone rather than down a Zone.

> It is better to apply an Amber Zone solution to a Green Zone problem; than it is to try and apply a Green Zone solution to an Amber Zone problem.

This simple tactic applies to all the different types of problems that you may experience and want to deal with.

We will use The Stepping Stones approach to understand, work with and then achieve the outcomes that we want.

This simple process can help you achieve positive results again and again.

The Stepping Stones that you can use again and again are:

1. Preparation & Practice.
2. Tackling the problem, issues or challenge.
3. Moving on and consolidating.

Just like with your weight problem; if you fall off a Stepping Stone, you simply begin the process again and learn from falling off the Stepping Stone.

And just like I suggested with your weight problem; you can take baby steps and you can tackle any problem by degrees.

If you make a mistake and get things wrong; then simply do what I told you to do with your weight problem. Use failure to show you what you need to do to achieve success.

So all of this becomes a simple process that you can incorporate into your life and it is simple to follow.

It will not always be easy but by being consistent you can achieve positive results that you never thought you would be able to achieve.

In Summary

To lock things in place and to continue moving forwards in a positive way, we can use the 3 Stepping Stones approach combined with The Dieters Scale, to help us achieve and succeed with our Positive Lifestyle Management.

The Dieters Scale helps up to understand the size of the problem. Is it a small Green Zone problem? Is it a medium size Amber Zone problem or is it a large Red Zone problem.

If you classify it in the wrong Zone it is not a problem; simply move it into the right Zone when you realise it and then start the process from the beginning.

It is better to go a Zone up than it is to go a Zone down.

As you move on to the 3rd Stepping Stone you might be expecting me to give you some sort of Secret. In reality the Secret is that there is no Secret.

You can benefit from the thousands of hours of work that have gone into creating The Human Algorithm® Approach to resolving, improving and better managing problems.

What there is in this book and the work that I do, is great design and implementation of a strategic solution to weight problems.

You can benefit from this by keeping this book with you and reading through it again and again as you improve and then master your weight problem.

As you come across other people with weight problems, you can point them towards this solution and allow them the opportunity to help themselves into a better future.

CHAPTER 28

Creating Your Slim Land Identity

Well, we are moving towards the end of this book but not the end of the wonderful things which you and I can create and achieve.

Regardless of how difficult, complicated or bad life gets; life is a golden opportunity that we need to take and enjoy.

To help you with this I am going to give you another piece of the dieters puzzle.

If you are someone who has a weight problem, a number of things would have changed in your life as that weight problem developed and became established.

Your life profile will have changed.

Our life profile changes as we move through life and as we grow older. An example is someone who trains to become a professional and they become known for being someone good at that work.

This might be a plumber, a carpenter, an accountant, etc.

These are example of our work or professional identities.

As well as developing a professional or work identity we also develop a personal identity; one that our family and friends know us by and one that we know ourselves by.

For example: That slim, elegant and confident person who lives down the street.

I think that many people with weight problems also take

on an identity and that is their Fat Land Identity.

Their Fat Land Identity begins to define who they are, what they do, how they do it, what you can expect from them and how they respect and value themselves.

Now at this point I know that there are some people who will want to give me an argument about this.

I have noticed that there is a trend for people saying that we should not recognise or see someone's weight; in the same way that we should not see or recognise the colour of someone's skin.

"We should see the person inside."

My view on this is simple!

I have not come across many people who have weight problems who are really and genuinely happy with being overweight; with the effects and affects that this has upon themselves and the lives that they have.

I have come across a lot of people who begin by claiming that this is the case, but when we have got beneath the surface the rhetoric changes.

If you want to be overweight and live a happy life I don't have a problem with that. I am not going to waste a single breath telling you any different.

I am interested in the people who are not happy having a weight problem and who want to really do something about it, so that they can feel better about themselves and have happier and more fulfilling lives.

So let's get back to those people who do want to change and improve their lives and leave the people alone who don't want to change and improve their lives.

As I said before:

Their Fat Land Identity begins to define who they are, what they do, how they do it, what you can expect from them and how they respect and value themselves.

Changing all of this is something that we do in baby steps and we began that process back in the first part of this book: Preparation & Practice.

With some things you will find that it is easy to leave your Fat Land identity behind and to embrace your Slim Land identity.

With other things it may be more difficult.

The things that are more difficult just require you to do them in stages: Moving a little bit at a time.

One major reason people have a problem with the difficult bits is this:

> They shy away from changing or dealing with certain parts of the problem.

Now when you do this you are, in effect, trying to be in two place at once. You are trying to be in Slim Land but without leaving Fat Land.

The more that you try to do this, the more challenging and difficult it becomes. This then results in you having increased stress and things becoming more difficult and chaotic.

It is not unusual for someone to be taken back to Fat Land from their journey into Slim Land because of things like this.

I have helped people to finally move on and let go of their connections to Fat Land a number of times and it is always the same.

Once they have dealt with things properly and not compromised themselves; they can then move into Slim Land and begin to get to the right place in Slim Land for them.

The more time that you spend in Slim Land without having a foot in Fat Land the easier it will get for you.

Allow your weight to change, allow your life to change and allow yourself to change.

We continued with the baby steps approach when we moved on to the 2nd Stepping Stone: Diet & Weight Management.

We will continue with those baby steps as you consolidate your position and positive weight management becomes a part of your normal everyday life.

On the 3rd Stepping Stone you combine everything you have done so far and you continue to use The Dieters Scale and the 3 Stepping Stones Approach.

If you continue with this, then you will find that you gradually become established in Slim Land.

You will realise that life has changed and you may not quite realise exactly when it happened and how it happened; but it has happened.

You will find yourself in Slim Land and in order to stay there you just continue to do what you have done and use the same tools and processes that I have given you.

If you find that you need extra help at any time you can always send me an email to the address at the back of this book or through my website.

I think that for now, I have said everything that I need to say and I wish you well on your journey from Fat Land to Slim Land in 3 Steps!

HAVE A WONDERFUL JOURNEY!

About the Author

Life would be great if it was perfect. Unfortunately life often falls short of perfection and often lacks clarity.

How do we make a better life in an imperfect world with lots of competing pressures?

Nature provides us with a lot of gifts that we can use to experience Life and to help us to be successful in whatever environment that we find ourselves in.

Unfortunately these gifts do not come with instructions and we need to learn through experience how to understand, interpret and manage these wonderful gifts.

Nature does not provide us with instruction manuals but it does provide us with special people who are able to help us with living our lives and making our living experiences the best that they can be.

Guru David is one of these special people.

Why would someone want to use a Guru?

Guru's tend to live a different life to normal people. They have different life experiences and they think and behave differently.

Guru's will often have encountered and overcome many types of hardships and difficulties. These will often be physical and cerebral and can occur over long periods of time, often decades.

Guru's will understand Humanity and Human Nature better and they often have insights and understanding of things that others do not.

Guru's make good guides, advisors and mentors when difficult, complex and challenging issues have to be addressed. They provide confidentiality and support as appropriate and help to achieve clarity of thoughts and actions.

A good Guru deals with reality and understands societies structures and pressures.

Meet an extra ordinary person

Guru David creates custom approaches for challenges that involve Feelings, Emotions, Psychology, Behaviours, Experiences, Knowledge and acquired Wisdom.

Guru David accepts selected personal and business clients that he feels that he can work with.

Guru David's approach includes using The Way of Vartis and his authoritative work with The Human Algorithm® Project.

A graduate of The College of The Richmond Fellowship; an experienced counsellor and therapist with specialist training, knowledge and experience of Alcohol and Drug Addiction with a high level of knowledge and experience working with dependency issues, problem architecture, problem dynamics and related Human Algorithm's®.

Guru David is an authority on working with Obesity and Weight Control issues and provides a customised approach that includes work from his books covering this subject.

Due to his work with problem architecture, problem dynamics and Human Algorithm's, Guru David is well placed to understand many different problem types and provide help to develop effective solution focused approaches.

Guru David's other books include understanding Motivation; working with Self Esteem and The Human Dynamics Matrix.

Guru David's other experiences and knowledge include obtaining black belts in martial arts, experienced in working with finance and debt resolution for members of the public, business consultancy, different levels of training, writing books and articles, being targeted by trolls, being victimised and abused for having a different view and behaviours, being targeted and the victim of financial crimes, experience around the music industry, innovation, design, building and an interest in different types of engineering, construction, physics and nature.

At different times, Guru David's resilience has

inspired and amazed others and frustrated those who have tried to destroy him and his work.

Guru David has other knowledge, experiences and wisdom that can be revealed and shared at appropriate times.

Guru David would describe himself as spiritual rather than religious and this is evident in The Way of Vartis.

The Way of Vartis offers a view of the celestial reality of the universe, the truth about the future, the knowledge that people need to change how they live within their personal environments and the honesty of the reality of Life and why we are here.

The Way of Vartis provides an open approach and does not impose dogma. As a result someone can choose to add The Way of Vartis to their life and achieve the benefits without being required to give up any religious practices or beliefs they hold.

Guru David can be hired or consulted for specific or more general work.

Those who are interested in supporting The Way of Vartis or The Human Algorithm® Project can become a follower, supporter or sponsor.

Guru David can work in a variety of countries by arrangement and is comfortable to work through good quality interpreters.

Hello Readers!

You can find more information about the things that I am doing by visiting the following websites:

www.gurudavid.co.uk

www.vartis.co.uk

You can email me; Guru David with any comments or inquiries at: david@gurudavid.co.uk

Our Intellectual Property includes the following which is protected by Copyright, Trade Marks, Registered Trade Marks, Design Rights and Trade Secrets.

The Human Algorithm® Project

The Human Intelligence (**Hi**) Common Platform

The Dieters Scale and its various concepts and applications

The **Hi**-Way Stepping Stones Approach

The Fat Land and Slim Land concepts

The Fat Land and Slim Land Identity concepts

The Slim Land Quest & The Stepping Stones Quest

The 3 Steps Approach to dealing with the Weight Control problem and the different Common Components.

The Common Components, the Basket of Common Components, the Spiders Web

These were created and developed by Guru David aka David John Sheridan – Lifestyle Services Corporation Ltd (UK)

www.ingramcontent.com/pod-product-compliance
Lightning Source LLC
Chambersburg PA
CBHW072222270326
41930CB00010B/1952
* 9 7 8 0 9 9 3 2 3 5 5 2 8 *